FIT FOR COMBAT

By
JD Johannes, USMC

With
Nita Marquez,
IFBB Professional Fitness Competitor

Published by Red Vermillion, Topeka, Kansas, U.S.A.

The information provided in FIT FOR COMBAT should not be construed as a health-care diagnosis, treatment regimen or any other prescribed health-care advice or instruction. The information is provided with the understanding that the authors and publishers are not engaged in the practice of medicine or any other health-care profession and does not enter into a health-care practitioner/patient relationship with its readers. The publisher does not advise or recommend to its readers treatment or action with regard to matters relating to their health or well-being other than to suggest that readers consult appropriate health-care professionals in such matters. No action should be taken based solely on the content of this publication. The information and opinions provided herein are believed to be accurate and sound at the time of publication, based on the best judgment available to the authors. However, readers who rely on information in this publication to replace the advice of health-care professionals, or who fail to consult with health-care professionals, assume all risks of such conduct. The publisher is not responsible for errors or omissions.

CONTENTS

Part I From Fit (Enough) for Combat to Fit for Combat

Part II Fit for Combat System

Part III: The Road Forward

Part IV: Women and This System

Appendices

INTRODUCTION
by J.D. Johannes

Fitness is a matter of life and death for me.

I am not a personal trainer. I am not a model. I am not a certified by any exercise science organization. I have not and probably will not compete in a bodybuilding contest.

I am a regular guy with a job that requires an extraordinary level of physical conditioning. My job? I make television shows and documentaries in Iraq and Afghanistan.

As a former Marine and now a combat cameraman, I know from first hand experience what kind of strength and conditioning it takes to run around Iraq and Afghanistan with Army Paratroopers, U.S. Marines & Special Forces Teams while wearing body armor, a Kevlar helmet, carrying a gallon of water and a fifteen-pound television camera.

Like I said, fitness is a matter of life and death for me.

My training for function in the sands of Iraq and the mountains of Afghanistan—strength, speed, power, endurance—is also the most straight forward workout and diet system for regular people who want to look good on a sandy beach.

But it is not just for guys. This system is awesome for women and parts of it were designed for me by a woman—International Federation of Body Building Professional Fitness Athlete Nita Marquez, who competes in contests where her physique is judged on muscularity, shape and definition and has to perform a high energy dance and gymnastics routine.

Before I met Nita, I was what I call 'Fit (enough) for Combat'. I had been to Iraq several times to shoot video for television shows and documentaries and functioned just fine—but I was carrying around more fat than I wanted to. I wanted to keep the muscle and stamina, but lose the fat.

With some very basic advice from Nita, hard work in the gym and simple changes in my diet, I became truly 'Fit for Combat'.

What you will find in this book may shock you. Shock you at the straight forward simplicity of the training and diet. It shocked me. Because as you will see, it was not that I needed to do anything more, I just needed to do it right and a lot of you may actually need to do less than you are right now.

This book is not about me or Nita telling you to do this or do that, eat this, but not that. This book is an explanation of how to use certain tools to find the workout and eating plan that works for you so that you can become your own diet and workout guru.

~ J.D. Johannes

FORWARD
by Nita Marquez

Being an elite level fitness athlete has not come easily to me.

There are a number of people who are born with great genetics, whose bodies either stay lean and agile or respond to any type of training. However, in the world that I live in, the fitness and bodybuilding world, there is a science, more accurately, a scientific method to what we do. Many of us set forth into this realm going against the grain fighting a daily battle against our own DNA. In other words, you would be surprised just how many people in bodybuilding and fitness are not genetically inclined to being as lean and/or muscular as we ultimately achieve.

There is a science to it, and that science, when employed properly, leads us to our own customized training and eating plans to build strength, muscle and lose body fat.

This brings me to JD. When I first met him he was a great big bear of a man at the peak of what he calls his "heavy duty phase." As an analytical person, JD had come up with quantitative tools and measurements that, even after years of competing in fitness, I had never encountered. He fully grasped the science of building muscle, power and strength. But he wanted to be leaner and lighter while still maintaining his strength and power. The problem was JD's genetics were predisposed to keeping him thick and bear like.

The point here is that there is a broad range of fitness goals a person could set out to achieve. Each one of us has our own unique DNA. Which puts each of us into our own unique category as to what type of workout program and eating program will achieve the goal. Each person will have their own path to achieving their goals, but that path will still follow the science.

In this book you will read about JD's journey, the path he took to being lean, strong, powerful and with endurance and stamina to spare. Your path will probably not take you to a war zone, but the journey will take you to places within yourself. And if you stay on the path, your journey will bring you into the strength, leanness and stamina that you so desire.

The key is not duplicating every step in someone else's journey. It is in finding your own path by learning from the observation (not duplication) of another's path.

I am quite certain that if you are reading this book, you yourself have been going against the grain as well and been fighting a difficult struggle against your own DNA. You have tried everything the magazines told you to do, and you have voraciously followed instructions from every DVD or website you could get your eyes on. But the truth is, the answers are already in you. You just need to know and apply the scientific method to find the answers.

What JD and I hope to accomplish with this book is to explain the scientific method I used, he used and countless other physique athletes have used on our journeys. And that is the beauty of this. Though we all have different paths and journeys, though we all have different goals and DNA, the same scientific method can be used by all of us.

~ Nita Marquez

PART I

FROM FIT (ENOUGH) FOR COMBAT TO FIT FOR COMBAT

CHAPTER ONE
THAT GUY

"I need to be lighter," I thought to myself as I climbed yet another wall and dropped down onto the hard packed sand.

I was in Kharmah, Iraq on patrol with a squad of Marines. Their patrolling technique wasn't to drive around in Humvees, or walk down the roads and alleys of this dusty city by the Euphrates river—no, these Marines jumped over walls and jumped roof-top-to-roof-top.

I was 32-years-old and weighed 240 pounds. Throw in the body armor, Kevlar helmet, water and a 15 pound camera and I was having to move almost 290 pounds. To top it all off, it was 105 degrees in the shade. I really needed to be lighter.

I couldn't lose any of the body armor or gear, but if I lost 20 pounds of fat, that would definitely make the work of chasing around young Marines a lot easier.

Thirteen years earlier, I was a young United States Marine. I could do 20 pull-ups, run three miles in 20 minutes and do 80 sit-ups in two minutes. I weighed in at a whopping 170 pounds.

After I left the Marines and started working in television news, I quit running, but kept lifting weights. I was stronger and in better shape than my new civilian peers and for the next decade, that was good enough for me.

When the war in Iraq started, I was still a weight lifting guy, but once I knew I was going to be going to Iraq with my old Marine Corps unit to make a documentary of their deployment I went back to combat training—weights, distance running and sprints.

I did three tours in Iraq being 'Fit (enough) for Combat'. The key to me being 'Fit (enough) for Combat' was a very simple weight lifting system and a notebook. And I cannot stress enough the importance of the notebook.

It was the notebook that was the key ingredient to making me 'Fit (enough) for Combat' and then truly, 'Fit for Combat' and the foundation of this training system.

But it took me years to learn it's importance.

Before the notebook, I was *that guy*. We all see him at the gym, going through some insane workout he found in a glossy muscle magazine. This week he's doing the 'Armageddon Arm Workout'. Next week he'll be doing 'The Hulk's Huge Chest Workout'. For years I was *that guy*.

We all see him at the gym. I was him. A lot of people are him. Being *that guy*, can be a good thing. If a person has the guts to do the Armageddon Arm Workout with six different biceps exercises, for five sets at 20 reps each—they have what it takes to be 'Fit for Combat'.

That was me for seven years. I did every crazy workout of the pro-bodybuilders, every crazy diet and took every brand new supplement that was advertised. But nothing really worked.

When I was discharged from the Marines, I was 5'10" and weighed 170 pounds. After seven years of going to the gym and lifting weights four or five days a week, I was up to 205 pounds and 15 pounds of that was fat.

But I still kept doing 'The Hulk's Huge Chest Workout'. I still kept doing the 'Armageddon Arm Workout', but all I got was really sore.

I started imitating the workouts of some of the bodybuilders in the gym. I watched them closely, doing their exact same routines. Unfortunately for me, those were even less successful than the workouts in the glossy muscle magazines.

At the time, all I wanted to do was look good—maybe even look like a bodybuilder.

The mistake I constantly made, was emulating a guy who already had a champion physique, instead of doing what he did a couple years or even a decade earlier to get the champion physique.

It is a common mistake. Which can be, in many ways, a good thing. If a person has the guts to go through those workouts, and stick with it despite minimal gains, they are ready to take it up a notch. Or, as I discovered, down a notch.

All of those years I had the desire, dedication, and guts to keep at it. However I didn't have the knowledge. By just showing up and putting in the work, I was 70%

of the way to where I wanted to be. Most people who are dissatisfied with their appearance or condition do not even show up at the gym and work hard.

I showed up consistently and put in the effort, but the effort was not getting me what I wanted.

Over the course of all those years, when I was *that guy*, I showed up and put in the effort. I did what the bodybuilders did. However I missed an important step. I should not have been doing what they were doing now, or what took them from a State Champion to a National Champion. I needed to be doing what took them from where I was to a guy who actually looked like a bodybuilder.

Shaving my legs, chest, arms, etc., painting on a tan, getting oiled up and posing on a stage in a man-kini is something I have no desire to do. I have no desire to be a competitive bodybuilder. But like a lot of guys, I wouldn't mind looking like I could (not just telling myself that I could).

Most people will never have to be in good enough shape to run around Iraq in full body armor, vaulting walls, jumping roof-top-to-roof-top, but if you are in good enough shape to do it, you will look good in a pair of swim trunks at the beach.

It took me a long time to figure out how to move beyond being *that guy*.

The first step for me was to acknowledge that I needed to change. I needed to change my mind-set. When I fully embraced the fact that I wasn't making any progress, but knew I had the desire, dedication and guts—I was ready to take the next step.

――――――――――――― CHAPTER TWO ―――――――――――――
ADMITTING YOU HAVE A PROBLEM

My awakening occurred in the Fall of 2001. It must have been similar to an addict realizing he had started an irreversible slide. I finally admitted I was chasing something that couldn't be found in the glossy muscle magazines. I was coming clean, so to speak, with reality.

This isn't to say glossy magazines are bad, you can learn a lot from many of the articles. The problem was, I wasn't learning, I was imitating. When I finally realized that, I started down a new path.

Seriously. It was almost like saying, "My name is JD Johannes, and I'm that guy. I've been busting my ass in the gym, taking all the expensive supplements, doing all the crazy workouts, but I'm still not making any real progress."

Why it took me that long…I don't know. Pride, ego, stupidity, the general nature of humans…it doesn't matter.

But it took me seven years.

Here is an actual workout that I did back then:
  • Biceps--
  • Barbell Curls x 3 Sets
  • Dumbbell Curls x 3 Sets
  • Machine Preacher Curls x 3 Sets
  • Hammer Curls x 3 Sets
  • Concentration Curls x 3 Sets

No 205 pounder with 16-inch arms has any business expecting results from that workout. But I did it. I cobbled it together from the glossy magazines.

What I ate was even worse:
  • Breakfast—Meal Replacement Drink
  • Mid-morning—Sandwich
  • Lunch—Sandwich
  • Afternoon—Meal Replacement Bar
  • Evening—Sandwich
  • Night—Sandwich

Sometimes it was even more ridiculous. One Summer I would lift in the afternoons before going to work the swing shift, then come home and go for a run after work. Sounds like a good idea, right? But what did I do after my run and before I went to bed? I ate a big bowl of cereal. Eating all those carbs before I went to bed was really stupid.

Clearly, I had some odd ideas about training and diet—but I was always willing to put in the work. And after years of not seeing the results I wanted I was frustrated.

In my late-twenties, as my knowledge of economics, mathematics and philosophy expanded, I became more analytical in my approach to everything. I started applying those analytical tools to my work in the gym as well.

The workout routines and diets in the magazines are often cookie cutter advice. The magazines are read by thousands of people and therefore have to offer basic advice relevant to thousands of people. Those articles are designed for the so-called average person, or average weight lifter—but there is no such thing as average. We are all a little different and need different workout programs and eating plans to meet our goals.

I needed to take the time to find what worked best specifically for me. You will need to find what works specifically for you.

My quest for knowledge wasn't easy. Fortunately I stumbled into a guy who used to be a successful bodybuilder and he said something that really stuck with me, "Don't do what I do now, do what I did when I looked like you."

Whoa. Mind blowingly, simple advice. He went from ordinary to extraordinary with basic, simple, heavy workouts eating lots of protein and keeping a detailed training log. He explained how through keeping a detailed training log I would find what worked for me.

At first, I didn't want to believe it. It was too simple. Too straight forward. And not what I had been reading in the glossy magazines. So, I asked a few other 'big guys' how they did it. The advice was basically the same. But like any addict, I still resisted. However, I needed to be honest with myself—the other workouts and diets were not working, why not try this.

The hang up that held me back was the weight lifting program at my high school, which was the weight lifting program for the football team.

I was a decent player from a small school. When there are only 120 kids in your school, you are almost forced to be a letterman by your sophomore year.

The coach made us log our weight workouts. Like most kids, I rebelled. Years later, when it was suggested to me that I needed to start keeping track of my workouts, I dragged my feet. But I knew it was what I needed to do to reach my goal.

It was a great big power lifter turned bodybuilder that flipped the switch for me. He said, I should try to do more weight or more reps every time I came to the gym.

I had heard that advice probably a dozen times before from an old football coach of mine and decided to finally put the advice into action.

—————————————— CHAPTER THREE ——————————————
ROSENFIELD PRINCIPLE

Coach Rosenfield was the prototype old-school football coach. If you were to make a movie and needed an old school, bent nose coach, Rosenfield was who you would base the character on. A World War II veteran, tattoos on the forearms, bent nose, the works. Even in his 70s, when he would substitute teach phys-ed class, if you were a knucklehead to him, he could drop you with one punch.

But Rosenfield was also an intellectual. He played the stock market and commodities markets and had a broad portfolio of real estate. His degree was in education and biology and he always walked around with a book or two and a sheaf of research papers.

He coached right out the Bear Bryant school, but thought like a research analyst.

In weight lifting class, Rosenfield would say, "You have to lift more this week than did last week and lift more next week than you did this week." It would invariably be followed by a brief lecture on polynucleated cells.

After all those years, I was essentially hearing the same explanation again. To make the muscle grow, the key was to overload it week after week after week, overload the muscle over time.

It took me years to realize I already knew the secret to building muscle. Building muscle was not some fancy rocket science, but old school training backed by well established science.

All I needed to do was follow Coach Rosenfield's advice.

Admitting I had a problem was my first step to recovery. The second step was accountability. I started keeping a detailed training log. Every workout, every rep, every set, what I ate, the cardio, everything. After I started keeping a training log, I still resisted.

"I've seen that guy keeping a detailed training log," I would say to myself.

There are a lot of people who keep detailed training logs but never make any discernible progress. For them, the training log is more of an expression of a compulsive behavior than a training system. They write everything down, but they do not use the data they have collected.

This happens all the time in business. Information technology has allowed for a massive capture of data, but most of it just sits in digital reams, glanced at, stuffed in reports, but rarely analyzed. It is rarely analyzed because so few people understand regression analysis and linear programming, randomized testing, etc.

It reminds me of the Bill Lumberg character in the classic movie 'Office Space'. Everybody in the massive cubicle farm at a software company is writing and filling in their 'TPS reports'. So much effort was put into the weekly TPS reports they became an end unto themselves.

Reams of captured data are useless unless you use them. In the gym, I had to learn that the log book was not just about capturing data, it was a tool for analysis and to hold myself accountable.

A log book is invaluable. Without it you probably think to yourself, "Well, today is chest day, so I'll do bench." And you try to remember how much weight you did last time and how many reps you did. I did that for years. It doesn't work.

But even a training log will only take you so far if you do not use it correctly.

I had to use the data in the log book to apply the old-school Rosenfield principle—do more this week than you did last week, do more next week than you did this week.

The goal is to overload the muscles over time which induces continued muscular hypertrophy. The overload causes micro-trauma to the muscles. The little bitty tears and pulls in the muscle. The micro-trauma is what causes soreness in the muscle the next morning after a tough workout.

The body, when confronted with micro-trauma will do one of two things; increase the size of those traumatized cells (hypertrophy) or, rarely, increase the total number of cells (hyperplasia). Hypertrophy is the most common.

If the muscles are confronted with a greater load over time, the hypertrophy will continue over time, your muscles will continue to grow over time.

That can be accomplished through increased weight or increased reps. I found through trial and error that a progressive combination of increased weight and reps is what works for me. Coach Rosenfield knew it and explained it to us probably a dozen times back in that old musty weight room. But it never really sunk in until I started actually doing it. Do more weight or reps this week than you did last week, do more weight or reps next week than you did this week.

The notebook or the training log, then becomes a tool of accountability to set a target goal for Rosenfield's 'more'.

At this stage, I was like most serious hobbyists—confused. I was confused by the odd bodybuilding civil war between adherents of the various "reps" factions. In the magazines there are articles saying that heavy weights and low reps are the way to go. A few pages later there will be an article that says high volume, lots of reps are the way to go.

On the internet message boards the two camps wage daily battles arguing that 'their' method is the best.

In the end, I found it really doesn't matter. What does matter is the Rosenfield principle. Overloading the muscle over time works every time.

For the purposes of building muscle and strength, all that counts is overloading the muscle more this week than it was overloaded last week.

Before my wake-up call I would do bench press with 225 pounds for three sets. The first set I did ten, then eight, then six. Not bad, not great.

But I kept doing that every chest workout for months. I was not accomplishing anything because I was not increasing the overload. Because I never moved beyond 225 pounds for ten reps, then eight reps, then six reps. I was spinning my wheels. I was working the muscles, but I was not overloading the muscles over time.

I was still only doing 24 total reps with 225 pounds.

When I started using the log book to hold myself accountable, I started to build muscle again. I was following the Rosenfield principle of doing more this week than last week.

But my tracking system was tough to figure out. What exactly was the 'more' I should be doing each week? Did I want to increase the number of reps on every set or just the first one? If I got a lot more reps on the first one, it was harder to increase the number of reps on the next two sets.

I decided on a simple mathematical solution that adhered to the Rosenfield principle. I counted the total number of reps from the three sets.

The goal then became to do more repetitions over the course of three sets than I did the previous week on that exercise. It was a very straight forward approach until I got to where I was doing a whole lot of reps.

My solution was to increase the weight. That was a no brainer. I went for months increasing the weight rather arbitrarily. On some exercises I increased the weight after 15 total reps, on others after 30 total reps, but usually I just increased the weight when, I felt like I should increase the weight. Amazingly enough, it worked. The Rosenfield principle, over load over time works so well even if done in the most capricious fashion it still yields results.

After going through the hodgepodge of a few months of workouts I could see the trend, but there was no fixed measurement. I decided to make my target goal a fixed number of reps over the course of three sets.

Since, like most guys, I enjoyed moving big plates and big dumbbells, I picked a low number to be my target goal, my magic number—15. When I got to my magic number of 15 reps over the course of three sets, I increased the weight on that exercise. Fifteen seemed to work well for me because on the first set I would rarely get more than ten reps, which kept me using heavy weights, but not ridiculously heavy weights.

Here is a pretty typical example from when I first started keeping a log book of my workouts. Again, my magic number was 15.

Week #1
> Bench Press
> 235 x 8
> 235 x 6
> 235 x 3
> *Total Reps 17*

Week #2

    Bench Press
    240 x 6
    240 x 4
    240 x 3
    Total Reps 13

Week #3

    Bench Press
    240 x 8
    240 x 5
    240 x 3
    Total Reps 16

Week #4

    Bench Press
    245 x 5
    245 x 3
    245 x 2
    Total Reps 10

The tracking became rather simple when I stuck to a target number of reps—or my magic number of 15. I increased the reps or weight every week. By writing it down, I held myself accountable to get more reps every week. When I got to my magic number, I increased the weight by five pounds until I got to 15 reps over the course of three sets.

What I was doing was overloading my muscles over time. Not just overloading them on one exercise, or one 'burn out' set, but increasing the overload every workout over the course of weeks and months. I haven't stopped, so you could say I have been overloading over the course of years now.

For years I thought that if I wasn't really sore the next day, I didn't work out hard enough. But, being really sore may be a sign of excessive micro-trauma. If there are too many itty-bitty tears and strains on the muscle, the body has to put all its energy and nutrients into getting back to where it was before the trauma. This is commonly referred to as over training.

A lot of people, myself included, make the mistake of using soreness as the measure of a good workout.

The micro-trauma from the overload is a component in muscle growth. The key to the overload over time is the micro-trauma over time. More accurately, the micro-trauma a person can recover from and grow from over time.

I was overtraining for years. The 'Armageddon Arm Workout' is a prescription for extreme soreness and over training.

When the body is working overtime just to get back to the pre-overload, pre-trauma normal, it will not have much left over to grow. All that is required for hypertrophy is to get to an overload that causes micro-trauma.

To get to that overload and micro-trauma a person can recover from is the key and it is different for every person. This is where my pursuit of quantifiable measurements came into play. Through the use of the notebook I could quantify strength gains, but how could I quantify muscle gains?

This was a real Rosenfield type of question. The solution it turned out was high school geometry and the mathematical constant of Pi.

I could track the increase in size up my upper arm with a cloth tape measure, but how could I track the increase in muscle in my upper arm? I needed a way to control for the constant and two variables involved. The circumference, meaning the distance around the upper arm is determined by three things: Muscle, bone and fat. The size of the humerus bone is pretty much constant while the amount of muscle and fat can change.

I couldn't find a way to measure the volume of the muscles at home, but measuring the thickness of fat could be done with a set of body fat calipers. That is when it hit me.

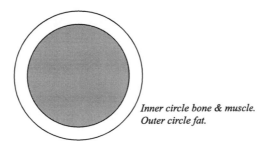

Inner circle bone & muscle.
Outer circle fat.

Think of the inner circle as muscle and bone and the outer circle as representing the layer of subcutaneous fat.

Using a cloth tape measure, I could determine the circumference of the outer circle. Using a pair of body fat calipers I could determine the thickness of the fat around the muscle. From there, it is geometry—Circumference divided by Pi equals diameter, subtract the thickness of fat and you know the lean tissue diameter. After a few practice runs I found it was best to do conduct these measurements with millimeters.

Back then, this is what the equation looked like:

Circumference: 394 mm
Fat Thickness: 4 mm

$394/3.14 = 125.47 - 4 \text{ mm} = 121.47 \text{ mm}$

The lean muscle diameter of my upper arm was 121.47 mm. Today, as I write this, my lean muscle diameter is 137.8 mm. That is a 16 mm increase. That may not seem like a lot, but back then my arms were a soft 15.5 inches, now they are a leaner 17.25 inches.

Keeping track of the changes in lean muscle diameter gave me a standardized, quantifiable way to track actual muscle gains and eventually find the precise workouts and overload that worked for me. What worked for me was failure, taking the exercise to the point I could not perform another repetition.

In the bench press example I used, the failure was in each of the three sets—which will cause plenty of micro-trauma. By increasing the number of reps and amount of weight over time, there will be micro-trauma to the muscles every time. Probably not a lot of soreness, but excessive soreness is a symptom of excessive micro-trauma.

To keep the micro-trauma and hypertrophy going, the muscles have to be overloaded over time. But what happens when you can't increase the number of reps or weight?

That was an important and difficult step for me, I had to learn to give up what I loved.

——————————————— CHAPTER FOUR ———————————————
BREAKING ADDICTION

I loved doing dips. Weighted dips, with 45-pound plates chained to my waist.

I got my first weight set when I was 12-years-old. The old sand-filled plastic weights from a discount department store and a bench. I set it up in the backyard near two large piles of cinder blocks.

In the muscle magazines I saw pictures guys doing dips and started doing dips on those stacks of cinder blocks. Over the years dipping became my best exercise. I could rep them out with body-weight as a teenager and was the first guy in high school to do them with a 45 pound plate strapped around my waist.

As I got older and stronger I kept doing them. They were my core upper body exercise and they are a great exercise. Truly, dips are the upper body version of the squat. But it got to the point that I could never move beyond 11 or so reps with three plates chained around my waist.

But I didn't care, I thought it was awesome that I could do it.

The problem was that all those years I did dips, with the same weight, with the same reps, I wasn't making any progress. I was wasting my time doing those dips. But I loved them and didn't want to give them up.

I was addicted to an exercise I was really good at. But, being good at an exercise is not what delivers progress. And just like the addiction problem earlier, I had to recognize that I was addicted, that I was not making progress and I had to be accountable.

When I acknowledge that I was addicted to dips, it made it easier to start giving up the comfortable exercises I was really good at in the pursuit of something bigger. Bigger muscles.

I was a dip junky. I was strung out on dips for years.

Everyone has their exercise. It's the one exercise for whatever reason, you're really good at. Humans tend to enjoy things they are good at. Since I am human, and was really good at dips, I enjoyed doing dips. But they were no longer rewarding me all those years of faithful service.

I had to get out of my relationship with dips. It was a tough one to break—but once I did, it was easier to break other hang ups with certain exercises and keep on the track of overloading over time.

Now, when I get to a point that I am not increasing the weight or increasing the number of reps on any, and I mean any exercise, I unsentimentally move on to another exercise for that muscle or group of muscles. That keeps the overload over time moving forward. Doing the same weight, for the same reps week after week is the anti-thesis of the Rosenfield principle of doing more this week than last week.

After overcoming my addiction to dips, I had to confront another hang-up.

I had always been enamoured with isolation exercises. And they have their place, but my gains from the Rosenfield principle, overload over time, did not take off until I went all the way back to the basics. Really, I can't imagine Rosenfield doing an isolation exercise, but for the longest time I still did them.

CHAPTER FIVE
BIG LIFTS

Dumbbell kick backs.

Not as addictive as dips, even more useless most of the time.

I was really going to add some 'shape' and bring out 'the detail' of my triceps by doing dumbbell kick backs. I saw a couple guys who competed doing them and thought, "Hey, if they are doing dumbbell kickbacks, I should do them."

Wrong.

I didn't need 'shape' or 'detail' in my triceps. I needed to get triceps first. As in discernible muscle size. Ninty-percent of how a muscle will look when fully developed is a function of DNA. I don't know what my triceps will look like when fully developed because even after years of overloading over time, they are still not fully developed.

So, I ditched all the 'shaping' and 'detail' exercises. They will have their place as isolation exercises to help bring a lagging body part, like if the delts dominate the triceps/biceps arms, but at this stage, I recognized the last thing I needed to worry about was balance and symmetry. Proportion, balance and symmetry are for bodybuilding competitors—I was a long way away from that.

It was another that guy realization. That guy wastes time 'shaping' a muscle that is not even close to fully developed. I realized I need to develop the muscle.

What adds big muscle? What would Rosenfield do? Big lifts. Bench, incline, rows, power pulls, barbell curls, shoulder press.

What I discovered was, I didn't have to do a whole lot of them. In fact, the fewer exercises I did, more muscle I gained. I made my biggest gains with two to three simple workouts.

This is a sample of what I did when I really started packing on muscle and strength. It came straight from Coach Rosenfield:

WORKOUT #1 UPPER BODY
- Dumbbell Shoulder Press
- Incline Bench 45 degrees
- Pull ups
- Cable Rows
- Barbell Curls
- Skull Crushers

(Three sets of each exercise to failure)

WORKOUT #2 LOWER BODY
- Squat
- Leg Curls
- Toe Risers
- Shrugs
- Abs

(Three sets of each exercise to failure.)

Here is what a couple weeks rotation looked like:
- Monday Workout #1
- Tuesday Low Intensity Cardio (LIC) (Treadmill 4 mph on an incline)
- Wednesday Workout #2
- Thursday LIC
- Friday Workout #1
- Saturday Off
- Sunday Off
- Monday Workout #2
- Tuesday LIC
- Wednesday Workout #1
- Thursday LIC
- Friday Workout #2
- Saturday Off
- Sunday Off
- Monday Workout #1

Mind numbingly straight forward. But what was the workout really doing? There is nothing magical about it, except that it caused frequent micro-trauma from the overload that was easy to recover from. It struck a real balance between frequency of trauma, the itty-bitty tears and strains, and the time to recover from the trauma.

I let this rotation run for a few months until the strength gains started slowing down and the increases in the lean muscle diameter in my upper arm slowed down as well. This workout was no longer working and I could determine it was no longer working with quantifiable evidence.

In the past, when confronted with a plateau I would make some radical changes. I would find a new workout in a magazine or on-line and try it. But that is like rolling the dice. The odds of picking the right workout for me are like shooting craps at a casino. So, instead of rolling the dice, I changed one of the variables, the frequency of the workouts.

I experimented with a little more advanced rotation as follows:

- Monday #1
- Tuesday LIC
- Wednesday #2
- Thursday LIC
- Friday #1
- Saturday LIC
- Sunday #2
- Monday LIC
- Tuesday #1
- Wednesday LIC
- Thursday #2
- Friday LIC
- Saturday #1
- Sunday LIC
- Monday #2
- Tuesday Off
- Wednesday Off
- Thursday #1
(Repeat the Pattern)

This rotation didn't seem to work as well for me. After a few months my strength crept up a little, but there was a slight decrease in my lean tissue diameter. Something was wrong with this workout.

It created a frequent pattern of micro-trauma to the muscles, but did not allow enough recovery time for maximum recovery—the hypertrophy, building back the muscle cells larger than they were.

Through tracking the workouts in my log book and the lean muscle diameter, I determined that an increase in frequency was not what I needed. So, I decreased the frequency.

I decided to try the old reliable three exercises, three times a week.

Monday Workout #1
• Shoulder Press
• Bench
• Skull Crushers
(Three sets to failure.)

Wednesday Workout #2 Legs
• Squat
• Leg Curls
• Toe risers
(Three sets to failure.)

Friday Workout #3
• Lat Pull downs
• Barbell Curls
• Shrugs
(Three sets to failure.)

My strength started going up and the lean tissue diameter started increasing again. My body needed more time to recover and fewer overall exercises to induce the over load needed to make my muscles grow.

What I discovered over the course of my first year of keeping a training log and holding myself accountable to do more this week than I did last week is that the individual

NITA SPEAKS _____

Micro-trauma and overload is **necessary for growth,** along with the three other very obvious components to muscle growth: **rest for recovery, proper nutrition, and supplementation**. Issuance of micro-trauma to the muscles comes through increase in weights or reps. How does one know when to increase? If you're working out effectively, you should have increases to workload (and thus, to strength capacity) every workout wherein you have availed the appropriate nutritional intake and rest to a muscle group.

In other words, **challenge your strength capacity** to the point of micro-trauma (usually, you will have a soreness by the end of each set as a note of your capacity). **Eat right** after with the correct nutrition and supplementation (*note, some supplementation may be ingested prior to the workout as well as right after and even throughout the rest of the day/night). Ingest an appropriate amount of **water** throughout your workout, and throughout each day. **Rest** at least a week, for allowance of proper recovery and development availability to the muscle group. Repeat ad infinitum.

This cycle always results in muscle growth, increased strength capacity, assists in dissolving fat, and therein, **increases stamina.**

exercises I chose did not matter. The rotation and exercise order really didn't matter as long as it was consistent for purposes of tracking. What counted was the overload over time.

Beating my total number of reps over the course of three sets until I hit the magic number is what worked. It does not matter what the magic number is, which is why I started calling it the magic number as a joke. There is no biological power in the number of reps. There is no secret number of reps that builds muscle. What builds muscle is overload over time that yields a level of micro-trauma the body can recover from. More specifically, the over load and micro-trauma my body could recover from.

When I hit a plateau of repetitions and could not get to my magic number, I quit doing that exercise. When I hit the plateau on flat bench, I moved to incline. When I hit plateau on incline, I moved to flat dumbbell bench. When I hit the plateau I moved on to something else working those same muscles. Eventually I came full circle back to flat barbell bench.

It was amazing. I was getting more out of three sets of basic, heavy barbell curls than I did out of six or eight sets!

Overload over time is an undeniable force. When you get to a point on an exercise that you cannot increase the reps or weight, replace that exercise with one that works similar muscles.

Even with as much as I had learned, or, more accurately, discovered through accident and trial and error, there was one element of my tracking that was off.

It was an element that made the tracking more precise and added an odd element to a very basic power/mass weight lifting system. My weight lifting was about to become a cardio killer.

--------------------------------- **CHAPTER SIX** ---------------------------------
A FAST WORKOUT

There he is, that guy who takes 90 minutes or two hours in the gym. He lolly gags between sets, has a conversation, wonders around, reads his glossy magazine.

I used to waste my time too.

To get through a bicep workout that I listed back in Chapter 1, it took me an hour. I would do a set, walk to the water fountain, lollygag around and wait until I felt I was 'recovered' enough to do another set.

I'm not exactly sure why I did it that way. Other than pride. I could do more weight, or, it was the only way I could get to around ten or eight reps on every set. Back then I still thought the number of reps per set had some magical value (which is why I now half in jest refer to the magic number).

My favorite version of that guy is the one who racks up six plates to do bench on the smith machine then takes an eternity between sets. I've gotten through entire workouts in the time it takes for him to do three sets.

When I first started paying attention to overload over time, I didn't pay any attention to the time between sets. Of course, that led to some wild variance from week to week. It was obvious my tracking was off. It is obvious that a two-minute break between sets will allow a person to do more reps than a one-minute break. If the tracking is off, the accountability is off and so is the overload over time.

Luckily the time between sets is an easy variable to control.

When I first started keeping track of time between sets, the gym I worked out at had a large digital clock in the weight room with hours, minutes and seconds. That made it pretty easy to look up and track one minute between sets.

When I changed gyms, I tried using a wrist watch, but it drove me nuts to have something on my wrist while lifting weights. So, I started doing something very simple. Old fashioned and low-tech counting breaths between sets worked well for me. Is it very accurate? No. But it's consistent enough to manage my tracking.

Keeping track of time between sets kept the tracking consistent.   It also added a little cardio element to my workout.

I started out with one minute between sets. That was pretty good, kept things consistent, but I wasn't 'winded' after three sets.

The next week, I tried 50 seconds. Still not winded.

After a few weeks I settled on 40 seconds. It was just enough to keep me breathing hard between sets. And viola. I added a cardiovascular element to a hard core mass and power workout and ditched all the low-intensity cardio.

It really doesn't matter what is used to measure time between sets. Breaths, seconds, sands through an hour-glass—just as long as it is consistent.

The next move was to quit lolly gagging between exercises. I started to move quickly, claim my area, rack the weight (which I knew I should be doing by looking back a few pages in my training log) drink some water and get busy again.

I was able to tear through these workouts in 30 minutes, tops. And I was worn out after 30 minutes.

That's it.

When I quit wasting time and started being consistent in the time I took between each set it added a nice cardio component. I ditched the low intensity cardio on the treadmill and started really packing on the strength and muscle.

I couldn't believe it at first. I was stunned. I had been conditioned to think that there is some complex secret, the magazines keep churning out articles of what the pros do and complex workouts. Something this simple, this straight forward couldn't be the solution.

It was.

During this process I had a few more mistakes to overcome. I was always willing to put in the work at the gym. I enjoyed lifting weights and therefore would gladly do lots of exercises. Lots of exercises should yield lots of results?

Nope. And that is the biggest mistake of them all.

CHAPTER SEVEN
WHY SAVE YOURSELF?

"You know, you could have done two more reps," my gym buddy Rob said after spotting me on military press.

"Yeah," I responded, "but I have four more shoulder exercises to save myself for."

Rob let out a chuckle, "You're saving yourself for lateral raises? What, are you going to marry the dumbbells? Are you saving yourself for your honeymoon with upright rows?" Rob said with a wry grin on his face. "Don't save yourself, take every set to failure and do fewer exercises."

Rob wasn't a really big guy. At that point my arms were a bit smaller than his, but he had a complete look. He was pretty lean all the time, and everything looked round and flowed well. It was a 'complete' look.

He kept all his workout results in a three-ring binder, and flew through his workouts taking every set to complete failure.

After really paying attention to his workouts, I never saved myself on one exercise so I could get through another.

But the problem was, I was still doing the 'Armageddon Arm Workout' taking a bunch of exercises, of five sets to near failure on every set. And the next week I would do some other hare-brained arm workout.

What was the difference between a guy like me and Rob? Rob was 35-years-old then and I was 27-years-old. He had found out what worked for him and could track and measure his progress, but he never got away from the basic principle of overloading the muscle.

When I was 'saving myself' for the rest of my workout, I was working the muscle, but I was not overloading the muscle. More importantly, I was not overloading it over time and tracking the overload over time.

A few times I spotted Rob at the gym.

"I need to beat 11 reps," he said, after glancing at his log book.

Rob wasn't trying to get 12 reps, or about ten to 12 reps. He had to beat 11 reps. Twelve reps was the minimum, but he wound up gutting through 13 reps and attempted 14.

I then asked Rob, "What would have happened if you didn't beat 11 reps?"

"I would have finished the exercise sets, going all out of course. And if my total number of reps didn't beat what I did last time, I would write 'DONE' next to it and the next time I worked my chest, would use a different exercise until I plateaued on it."

"How many times over the years have you plateaued on dumbbell incline?" I asked.

"At least a dozen. But every time, the plateau is at a higher weight," Rob said.

I bet Rob could dig through his old workout logs and show you exactly where he plateaued at. He would then come back to that exercise months or years later and would reach a new plateau.

Rob looks even better now than when I first met him. How many guys in the gym can say that? For the record, Rob was pushing 140 pound dumbbells. Pretty impressive for a guy in his early forties.

The key for Rob and a lot of people who have been successful in building muscle is overload. Overload every workout, every exercise, every set. Overload over the course of months and years.

Rob's DNA is not mine. He is not a naturally gifted bodybuilder. But he has through consistent tracking, accountability and overload, built himself into a dude who could seriously compete in a national masters competition.

Tracking your workouts in a log book, demanding of yourself to beat what you did last week is how you go from being where you are today to a guy like Rob.

CHAPTER EIGHT
THERE IS NO PLATEAU

There I was. I had my three ring binder, pen, bottle of water, simple workout, magic number, 20 breaths and every set to failure.

I felt kind of stupid at first with the three-ring binder. No, I felt really stupid at first with the three-ring binder.

I sheepishly wrote in it then stuffed it back in my gym bag. But something crazy happened when I started really overloading my muscles over time—I got stronger, a lot stronger. Stronger than I ever thought I could be.

After all those years of 'Armageddon Arm Workouts' I thought I had hit a stopping point, peaked, maxed out. I was wrong. I had not hit my body's genetic limit. I had hit the limit of what I could achieve through stupid workouts that were not dialed in on what worked for my genetics.

I hit the limit of what I now call casual progress.

Before I started really analyzing my workouts, I was working hard, but I was casual in my approach. I thought I had a workout plan, but it was not a long term plan. I thought I had a goal, but I didn't have metrics to measure progress toward the goal.

I thought I hit a plateau. I thought maybe this was all I had in me. I would see a workout like 'Plateau Breaking Pec Pump' in a magazine and give it a try. It didn't work.

At the time, I thought I was serious about working out—or at least a serious hobbyist. I was putting in time and effort, I wanted progress, but I was going about it very casually, very haphazardly. I thought a change up in workout would bust a plateau for me. That there was some silver bullet for breaking plateaus.

There isn't one. The only thing that breaks plateaus is to accept a plateau on an exercise and move on to another one, continuing the pattern of overload over time. Which means you can no longer be casual or haphazard about your workouts.

What I found when I started keeping the notebook, being accountable and overloading over time, is that I was able to make more progress with less overall effort. Three sets of arm curls to failure is really all I needed to stimulate muscle growth when I was overloading over time.

Additionally, when you are tracking your workouts and increasing the load gradually over time, you are no longer being casual. You may still be a hobbyist—but you now have a goal for every set of every exercise. Beat what you did last week, get to the magic number.

I'm no longer sheepish about my three ring-binder. People ask about it all the time, some people crack jokes, but the joke is on them. After months of overload over time, keeping the detailed training log I became a true believer. Every lift I did went up in weight to levels I had never encountered. I plateaued a few times, changed up exercises and took off again.

If you get only one thing out of this book, if you do only one thing I recommend, I hope it is keeping a training log and overloading over time.

After just a few months I was no longer stuck in a rut. I was making progress. I then applied the principles of tracking and keeping a notebook to something a lot of people forget. It's the one thing that is more demanding than the work in the gym. It's tracking what I put in my mouth.

CHAPTER NINE
FINAL FOUNDATION: FOOD

Every week was a new high for me after I started overloading over time and keeping a log book. I was getting stronger and building muscle. As I built more muscle my appetite increased. I was an eating machine. I ate. I mean I really ate, anything and everything in sight.

I ate chicken, steak, lunch meats, bread, pasta, meal replacement drinks, turkey, burritos, burgers, sub sandwiches, anything. I was getting stronger and there was a lot more muscle, but there was also a lot of fat growing around my waist.

A few extra pounds of fat didn't bother me at first, but then my pants started getting tight.

Then the gains in the gym started to slow down. I was still moving up in weight in lifts, but the increments were slower and the lean muscle diameter of my arm was at a stand still.

I was sold that the workouts and overload over time worked. So I turned my attention to my eating. I took a week and wrote down everything I ate, then calculated my protein, carbohydrate and fat intake.

At the time I was up to around 220 pounds, but only eating around 170 grams of protein a day. Even worse—some days it would be only 140 grams of protein.

Following the general rule of thumb from the magazines, I started consistently eating 220 grams of protein a day. Guess what, the strength gains started coming faster again and had a slight up-tick in the lean muscle diameter.

And something else happened, when I really started tracking my protein intake, it offset some of my carbohydrate intake—I stopped gaining fat. After a month my pants got just a little bit looser and I thought I had cracked the code.

In many ways, I had cracked the code. Overload over time, accountability, tracking, quick intense workouts, increased protein.

What I didn't know at the time was that I was laying a foundation for what was to come.

At this point in my life I was very happy to be a big muscular guy—being more muscular than my peers was all I wanted. Everyone else my age was starting to get a little more spread around the stomach. But my chest, shoulders and arms were slowly getting bigger and my waist stayed about the same size.

I continued down this path of overloading over time and making sure I got plenty of protein for three years. Then I made a decision. A decision that radically altered my life and ultimately led to this book, several documentaries, and TV shows. I decided to go to Iraq with my old Marine Corps unit.

CHAPTER TEN

FIT ENOUGH?

My heart was pounding out of my chest, my lungs were screaming, my legs were burning, I thought I might collapse.

I had only run .75 miles.

In December of 2004, I was sitting in the office my insurance agent, who was my old First Sergeant when I was in the Marine Reserve during college. We were shooting the breeze when he said the sentence that changed my life.

"You know, the Platoon is going to Iraq," he said. "They leave in a few months."

At the time I was an Assistant to the Attorney General in Kansas. Everyday I wore the political uniform of a suit or sports coat. Years earlier I had worked in television news as a photographer and producer.

Sitting in his office, I decided right then I was going to buy a TV camera and go to Iraq with my old unit as an embedded reporter and I would need to start getting in shape for combat.

The near heart attack inducing .75 miles run I took the next day showed me that I had to move from being a serious hobbyist about my training to treating it like a job.

I had a great foundation of fitness from all those years of overloading over time, but wars are not fought in a gym—they are fought on streets, open fields, on your feet.

Those first few runs were brutal.

My whole approach to training and eating changed. I was no longer trying to put on muscle to look better than my peers or because it was fun to be strong. Training went from a serious hobby to serious work.

I ratcheted up the intensity in the weight room and strength started accelerating. I kept my eating the same, with even more of a focus on making sure I got my protein, plus some more.

The major change was cardio. I started walking, then running on the treadmill. When it was warm enough, I would run outside. Those first runs outside killed me.

My workout rotation in preparation for that first trip to Iraq started like this:

- Monday—Weights
- Tuesday—Walking / Running
- Wednesday—Weights
- Thursday—Walking / Running
- Friday—Weights
- Saturday—Walking / Running
- Sunday—Off

The weight training was the old reliable three exercises, three times a week outlined in Chapter 5.

As the time for me to head to Iraq got closer, I increased the load:

- Sunday—AM Walking / PM Weights
- Monday—Running/Walking
- Tuesday—AM Walking / PM Weights
- Wednesday—Running/Walking
- Thursday—AM Walking / PM Weights
- Friday—Off
- Saturday—Sprints

My weight training was the basic three day workout:

- Sunday--Upper Body Push
- Tuesday--Legs, kinda light though due to all the running
- Thursday--Upper Body Pull

The walking started slow and I increased it by a few minutes every week. Toward the end I would power walk (sounds so like a housewife) for 45 minutes.

On the days I ran, I got up to two miles in 19 minutes then walked until I got to 45 minutes.

For the sprinting I did 100 yard sprints. I started slow, sprint 100 yards, walk 300 yards and gradually cut down the walking between sprints until I was sprinting 100 yards, then walking 100 yards and sprinting again for 100 yards. Right before I left I could do eight 100 meter sprint repetitions without dying.

The day came in March of 2005 for me to leave with the Platoon for Iraq. Whether I was 'Fit (enough) for Combat' would be tested soon.

CHAPTER ELEVEN
IN COMBAT

Boom. Boom. Boom. The artillery shells from the 155mm howitzers were fired from Camp Fallujah, sailed over our heads and impacted somewhere in front of us. We were driving at full speed toward where the shells were exploding.

Vengeance Platoon plus one embedded reporter was on its second mission.

Bait and Kill was the mission. I was with the bait element.

The platoon would drive up and down Highway 10 between Fallujah and Abu Ghraib in humvees with hillbilly armor. A few plates of steel and Kevlar pads duct taped to the doors. The goal was to get an insurgent cell to place a bomb on the side of the road. We were the bait.

The Kill element was a team of snipers who would hopefully shoot the insurgent cell before they blew one of our hillbilly humvees to pieces. It was during one of our thunder runs down Highway 10 that we heard the artillery shells impacting in front of us. We drove straight toward them into a fire fight.

Al Qaida in Iraq had launched a full scale assault on the prison at Abu Ghraib with rockets, mortars and suicide truck bombs. The Marines guarding the prison walls called in danger close fire missions from the 155mm howitzers to shred the waves of jihadists storming the prison.

Vengeance Platoon's new mission was to box in the insurgents and hunt them down house to house through the canal country near the Euphrates river. I would soon know if I was in shape enough to keep up with a bunch of 20-year-old Marines in combat. The red streaks of tracers flew over my head. Gunfire cracked in the darkness. "Contact at the warehouse," came the call over the radio.

The warehouse was 400 meters away through soft dirt and irrigation ditches. I jogged along side Lance Corporal Martin McClung and the ground pounders as the humvees bounced over the ditches. It was cool that night, but I was sweating under my body armor. So far the fast jog, even with all my gear wasn't winding me. But my load was about to get heavier.

One of the humvees hit a ditch hard with sharp clang of metal.

Some of the Platoon's humvees were equipped with TOW missile systems. The TOW, or Tube Launched Optically Guided Wire to Command link guided missile, was originally designed for taking out tanks, but in Iraq, where the insurgents used concrete houses like bunkers, the TOW punched holes through walls and solved a lot of problems. But when a humvee crashes into an irrigation ditch too fast, the missile tube will pop out of the breach.

I stumbled over the missile tube that popped out of the breach. Luckily the missile is relatively safe while still in the tube. But it weighs in at nearly 60 pounds and is almost four feet long. I bent down, picked it up and carried like I had seen TOW gunners carrying them years before when I was a young Marine in the School of Infantry at Camp Pendleton, CA.

The embedded reporter running along with the grunts was now an ammunition bearer. I ran for 200 meters like that until the humvee got into a firing position.

Some of the younger Marines, like McClung, were skeptical of me at first. The older guys in the Platoon remembered me from years before and vouched for me, but there were still questions. After I ran with a TOW Missile in my arms during a fight, all the questions were erased.

All the training had paid off. All the years in the gym as a hobbyist built a foundation of strength that allowed me to run with all my gear on, carry a TV camera and a TOW Missile.

All through the night and the next day we cleared houses. Up stair wells, over walls, across roof tops and I never missed a step. It was like that through the entire deployment. I never had a problem keeping up with Marines who were 10 years younger than I was.

One time as McClung and a few others were chasing down an insurgent, I was running so fast I got ahead of the Marines and had to slow down so I wouldn't be between them and the enemy.

My training system worked. It passed the ultimate real-life test. I was 'Fit (enough) for Combat'.

CHAPTER TWELVE
GETTING FAT IN IRAQ

Studies have shown the average soldier gains ten pounds while deployed to Iraq. I, not content with being average, gained closer to twenty pounds.

How does that happen?

Well, most soldiers and Marines never leave the wire. They spend their entire deployment on some huge base that is remarkably similar to a huge base in the United States.

These huge bases have what are called Dining Facilities or DFACs. The DFACs are better than any chain buffet style restaurant in the United States.

The food is good. Too good. And you can eat four huge meals a day.

The DFAC at Camp Fallujah is so good, it is nicknamed the Golden Corral. But personally I think the main DFAC at al Taqqadum is the five-star standard of military dining.

So there is the average soldier or Marine, putting in a 14 hour day working on Humvees, or fixing radios or whatever their job is and they get to eat four huge meals a day at a buffet.

But I spend two-thirds of my time with grunts, infantrymen who do their work outside the wire in the red zone fighting the war. Which leads us to the MRE or Meal Ready to Eat. In a plain brown plastic bag, the individual food items in sealed foil, guaranteed never to spoil and loaded with sugar and carbohydrates.

Eat three or four of those a day and you have the energy to compete in the Tour de France.

As physical as the work outside the wire is, it is not the Tour de France.

About one-third of my time is spent at a major base filing my news stories, logging tape and editing tape. I eat at the DFAC a lot.

On the second trip to Iraq in 2005, I arrived weighing 230 pounds. That is 230 with

18 inch arms and a 54 inch chest. When I arrived home I tipped the scales at 250.

Physically I was wreck. My left sciatic nerve, the one that runs from the lower back down through the glutes and hamstrings was acting up. Same with a nerve in my shoulder.

Mentally and emotionally I was exhausted. I took two weeks off to download before I started editing what would become my first documentary and getting back to normal life and training.

I knew another trip to Iraq would be coming and started building myself up again.

This time I used an A/B workout. In fact, the exact one outlined in Chapter 5 with a little more running and I ran sprints one day a week.

Over the course of a few months my strength was beyond my previous best. The lean muscle diameter was moving up and the fat was slowly coming off.

During this time the war was changing. Infantry units were spending more time on their feet and living in small combat outposts for months at a time.

I hit Iraq again for a long expedition, four months, in the spring of 2007. I had made a few milk-runs in 2006. Short two week trips on assignment, but those are just blips with little exposure to the daily grind of combat. This trip was going to be another test.

CHAPTER THIRTEEN
ANOTHER TEST

I was flying backward through the air.

A moment earlier I was standing around talking with a group of Army Paratroopers. Then a machine gun rattled 100 meters away.

The next thing I knew I was flying backward after being hit with a gust of wind and debris. Then I heard a sound that still rattles in my brain.

A suicide truck bomb loaded with more than 2,000 pounds of explosives blew up 300 meters from where I was standing.

An instant later the air was filled with the sound of gunfire. Combat Outpost Omar, a small building on the outskirts of a little village named Kharmah manned by two platoons of Army Paratroopers was under siege.

I had arrived at Omar late the night before. I was going to embed there because a large raid was about to be sprung on a neighboring village infested with Al Qaida fighters. This was not my first trip to Kharmah. In 2005, I rolled around the area with Vengeance Platoon as they hunted a notorious band of terrorists called the Green Battalion. The Green Battalion made their name by videotaping the decapitation of anyone they captured.

Kharmah hadn't changed much in two years.

As the melee ensued, I strapped on my body armor, grabbed my camera and looked for a way to get into the fight.

A group of sharpshooters were heading up to the roof and I thought to myself, "Yeah, that's where I want to be."

I asked if I could go with them and before anyone had enough time to say "no," Corporal John Hegland grabbed me. We ran out the door and up the stairs to the roof.

Hegland gave me a quick brief on the stairs. "The fires coming from over there," he pointed. "If you get between it, you're gonna get yourself killed. You ready?"

"Yep," I replied.

"One, two, three go!"

I followed him up the stairs and on to the roof.

I felt the breeze of a bullet fly past me then the unmistakable sonic crack. We were being shot at.

The first group of paratroopers heading to the roof may have caught the insurgents off-guard, but now they were waiting for us.

I dropped myself to the roof.

"In here, in here," he yelled scrambling into a sniper screen. The cloth wouldn't stop bullets, but at least they couldn't see us.

More shots rattled, Hegland and I stumbled over each other. I felt a burning sensation in my right knee.

We tumbled into the sand-bagged fighting position falling on top of each other.

"You just took fire!" Hegland exclaimed.

"I know. It's happencd before a few times," I said.

I looked down at my knee. A clean slice. The bullet just grazed me. The pain from a bullet wound in combat is the burn. The barrels of the machine guns are almost glowing hot and the rounds are super heated coming out. This bullet was so hot it almost cauterized the slice.

The paratroopers traded fire for 15 minutes. The mortar crew began launching shells from Omar into the insurgent's positions. Whomp. The mortar came out of the tube, a few seconds later, Boom.

Then it all ended. An hour later, the only evidence of the fight was the smoking hulks and craters from the truck bombs.

I crashed hard when the adrenaline was used up. We all swapped stories and watched some of my crazy roof run video until we could barely stand. That night I had the deepest sleep of my life. I was going to need it. The next day would a bring an arduous mission. The one I had been sent to Kharmah to cover.

Three kilometers east of Omar was Banana Town. A series of clusters of houses that arced like a Banana. Intelligence had indicated there may be surface to air missiles in that area. A missile had taken down a helicopter a few weeks earlier near Omar.

The U.S. Military loves to rule the skies and wanted to get those missiles out of the insurgent's arsenal.

The raid on Banana Town would start well before dawn. A multi-pronged attack, with platoons hitting each cluster of houses simultaneously.

The element of surprise was paramount. The route the paratroopers would use to get to the targets arced for almost five kilometers through the irrigated farm country.

We stepped off in the middle of the night, trudging quietly through the muddy fields and wading through the irrigation canals. In the east the moon rose and the planet Mercury hovered as a red dot above the horizon. The Greek god of war guiding the paratroopers to battle.

This was another test to see if I was 'Fit (enough) for Combat'. A five kilometer hike through mud and muck at night. The body armor was heavier than in the past with the addition of side plates. On my back was a one gallon Camel back. In my pack were some stripped down MREs and a second TV camera. The mission would transition from night to day and I didn't want to have to change lenses in the dust and dirt.

I was carrying a lot of gear, but some of the paratroopers were carrying even more.

Typical combat. Hours of walking, traversing terrain and when we got to Banana Town it became a series of sprints.

I flowed with the paratroopers in the entry stacks, following as they moved from room to room. As dawn broke they moved into the canal country. The dogs were on a scent trail. More mud and muck and canals to wade through.

I spent four months going at that speed.

I could keep up fine, but was sick and tired of carrying around the extra body fat.

The training had made me so durable that even during one mission when I was stricken with the dysentery I could still keep up with soldiers during a running gunfight in Baghdad.

I remember sending an email to a friend that when I got home I was going to do whatever it took to get down to a more reasonable weight.

What I found when I got back to the states was that as much as the overload over time had accidentally prepared me for combat a few years earlier, it had laid a foundation for something bigger, or should I say, leaner.

CHAPTER FOURTEEN
CRAZY IN MIAMI

"You're a big boy. And you have some figured out. Good," the French Canadian female bodybuilder said. "You are ready to start bodybuilding." Her French accent was thick and hard to decipher at times, but there was no mistaking she knew how to turn a person into a competitive bodybuilder.

I was down in Miami, visiting a friend from Iraq. He took me to the gym where his sister worked part-time and she introduced me to the crazy Miami Muscle Girls. The girls were a mix of Brazilians, French Canadians, Venezuelans and the rest of the United Nations of muscle.

When they looked at me, it was like a how a sculptor looks at block of granite.

At that time I was a big, strong guy. After years of constant overload, even with the trips to Iraq, I went from a soft 210 pounds to a soft 245 pounds. The whole time I kept the same level of body fat (at least visually it looked the same). There was always a 'hint of abs' at the top, but not much else.

If some people are built for show, and some are built for go—I was all 'go'.

As you have been reading, a lot of my work is overseas. It is in combat zones, where speed, explosive power and the ability to move over obstacles is paramount.

In addition to the basic mass/power workouts, I incorporated some sprints, plyometrics and agility/obstacle drills.

Heavy duty would be the best way to describe the way I looked—big muscles covered by a layer of fat. A 56-inch chest, 40-inch waist, 19-inch arms. In the gym I moved ridiculous amounts of weight. EZ curls with 180 pounds, dumbbell curls with 70 pounders. I mean seriously, a guy doing arm curls with 70-pound dumbbells looks absurd. But the absurdity was half the fun.

What wasn't fun was dragging 240-250 pounds around the villages of Iraq.

When I got home, my goal was to get down to 215 pounds while holding the same muscle mass. I figured 25 to 30 less pounds would make the work a lot easier.

What I didn't fully realize is that was carrying a lot more body fat than I thought—and I had no clue how to get rid of it.

When I got home, I put together what I thought would be a pretty good diet and exercise plan to lose some fat.

Here is a typical day from then:

- Wake up
- Whey Protein shake with Almond Milk
- Power Walk
- Meal #1 - Meal replacement shake
- Meal #2 - Steak, sweet potatoes, veggies
- Meal #3 - Meal replacement shake
- Lift weights or Sprints/Plyo/Agility
- Meal #4 - Meal replacement shake
- Meal #5 - Chicken, sweet potatoes, veggies
- Meal #6 - Steak or Chicken, sweet potatoes, veggies
- Meal #7 - Whey protein drink

The results after three months? Nada, nil, nothing. I just kept getting stronger and bigger. The lean muscle diameter of my upper arm kept going up. I was building muscle but also a lot of fat. I got up to 255 pounds at the peak.

I increased the duration of my cardio. Nothing. I increased the intensity of my cardio. Nothing. (I didn't know then that cardio can actually be a hindrance to fat loss. That will be covered later in Part II of this book.)

Then I found myself in Miami at the same gym as a group of insane women bodybuilders—the Miami Muscle Girls.

They were crazy, but they wcrc the best bodybuilders I have ever met. After knowing them I have come to believe that women are better at bodybuilding than men because they are more results oriented in appearance than men.

One of the crazy French Canadians, Lynn Suave, put me through the paces of a workout. She was impressed that I had my log book and a goal for each exercise. I had, on my own, discovered what they normally charge their clients a lot of money for—the system of overload over time.

The Miami Muscle Girls have what can best be described as factory churning out male bodybuilders, women bodybuilders, as well as fitness and figure competitors.

Since I already had the principle of overload over time down, and had built up a lot of muscle and a lot of strength they only had to teach me two things:

1. Super Intensity
2. How to eat

And when I say super intensity—I mean a whole new level of working out.

CHAPTER FIFTEEN
BLACKOUT WORKOUT

The room was spinning a little. I could hear people talking, music and weights clanging, but it sounded like I was underwater. All I could do was lay there on my back sprawled out on the black rubber mats of the gym floor.

A lot of people will collapse or vomit from a super intense leg workout. Ever heard of collapsing after a back workout? How about collapsing from a back workout of just four exercises that did not include dead lifts?

That is what I mean by super intensity.

Before I met the Miami Muscle Girls my magic number, the number of reps I set out to get over three sets was 15. I did well with 15.

A common set of barbell curls looked like this:

        EZ barbell curls
        180 x 7
               x 5
               x 3
        Total Reps 15

The Miami Muscle Girls thought that was good, but now it was time to crank things up a bit to say, 25 reps over the course of three sets or 30 reps over the course of four sets.

Of course the weight I used went down, but try this one on for size some time.

        EZ barbell curls
        135 x 13
             x 8
             x 5
             x 3
        Total Reps 29

Oh, and there was a strict 20 seconds rest between sets. They put me on a stop watch.

Every set to a bone crushing failure. The clock started at the first motion to put the weight down. And I had to have the weight in my hands and starting the next set at the 20 second mark.

After one of their shoulder workouts, I couldn't drive. I literally could not keep my hand on the steering wheel. I didn't even bother to try driving. I went back inside the gym, finished my protein drink and waited for 15 minutes until I could lift my arms again.

No 'Armageddon Arm Workout' had ever thrashed me the way those girls did over the course of just four exercises.

I am not sure I can adequately describe it with written words. The back workout I was the most brutal.

Cable low rows with a medium grip was the last exercise and I only did 190 pounds.

Set 1.
I hit the wall at 10 reps. On the 11th rep, I could only move it halfway, "Jerk it and hold it," she said sternly. So I did, and got it all the way to the top of the contraction then held it. "Keep the shoulder blades back," she said. So I did. "Down slowly," she insisted. It felt like forever. But I knew I wasn't done. Half reps were next, no arms, just pulling the shoulder blades together and trying to move my elbows backward while keeping my back straight up and down. When I couldn't even move the weight I was done with the first set.

That was 10.5 reps + 4 flails

> Set 2
> 6.5 reps + 3 flails.
>
> Set 3
> 3.5 reps + 2 flails
>
> Set 4
> A drop set to 140 pounds done just like set #1

It was like that when we started on wide grip pull downs, pull downs on a Hammer machine, dumbbell rows and then finishing off with cable low rows.

After the drop set on cable low rows I tried to stand up, but the thought of lying on my back on the floor seemed like a much better option.

"Now you know how to really train," she said looking down at me.

Once they determined I had the intensity in the gym, it was time get more intense on what really mattered—what I ate.

CHAPTER SIXTEEN

ABS LOOK BETTER THAN . . .

"Where's your cooler?" Lynnie asked as I walked out to her car.

My buddy from Iraq was pulling a shift in the emergency room and I was going to hang out with his sister, Lynnie, for the day. She doesn't compete in figure competitions or fitness competitions. She is a nurse and occasionally relaxes her diet, meaning she gets a little softer, to do Bikini Contests.

I explained I didn't have a cooler. And that began one of the greatest lessons I have ever learned on my way to becoming truly, 'Fit for Combat'.

She told me go back inside and grab my buddy's cooler, then we went to the grocery store, cooked and packed my cooler.

An hour later she was ready to show me all the sights of south Florida.

Lynnie told me if she is going to be out and around for a day, she takes her cooler packed with all her meals, whey protein powder, water. When she does a shift at the hospital, she brings it along as well. All her 'lunches' as she calls them. Nothing throws her off her eating plan.

Lynnie took me to a dance club on South Beach later that night. At 10:00 p.m. sharp we went back to her car to have a whey protein shake.

Was Lynnie obsessive? She doesn't think so. To her, stepping out of a dance club to grab a protein shake is the logical result of a choice. A choice to have six-pack abs year round.

"In my opinion, abs look better than anything tastes," she said. "I'll have something that tastes good on Saturday." On Saturday or Sunday she will have a cheat meal, usually something loaded with carbs followed by sweet dessert.

It was a Thursday, which meant fish, chicken, vegetables and sweet potato. She ate practically the same things six days week.

Her decisions are the crux of all economic decisions—a trade off.

The economist Thomas Sowell has a mantra—resources are scarce and have alternative uses, there is always a trade off and the market, the consumer, determines the value.

"I would love to be able to eat cheesecake and chocolate and still look this way," Lynnie said as we drove down the A1-A. "But I can't. Tight glutes and abs or cheesecake. No brainer for me."

Lynnie placed a higher value on her physique than she did the gastronomical pleasure of cheesecake and chocolate. The trade off was clear and she put a higher value on her physique.

Every bodybuilder, male or female, fitness competitor, figure competitor or person like Lynnie that I have met, eats five to nine times a day. Small meals, mostly protein, some vegetables and carbs without much sugar.

When eating like that many times a day, the cooler isn't just a necessity of the trade off, it is an unintended bonus of the trade-off. It is actually more convenient than how most people eat.

To understand the convenience, let me tell you about my friend Sarah. She is 29-years-old and was a serious hobbyist in the gym for years. She did the treadmill, elliptical and some weights.

She also has a career that makes her car her office—she is a sales representative for a medical technology company. Everyday she is making visits to doctor's offices, clinics and hospitals in her rather large and rural territory.

She recently decided to compete in the figure division of a small contest. I introduced her to Nita, who put her on a plan similar to what Lynnie does.

Sarah was going to have start packing a cooler as well.

"Before I would try to eat healthy, a chicken salad, a sandwich on whole wheat. It was easy to get a salad or a whole wheat sandwich just about anywhere. I thought the cooler was going to be real pain," Sarah said.

But, she wanted to follow the plan and started packing the cooler. She cooked a lot of her food ahead of time, weighed everything out and put it in the freezer. After a few days of packing her lunches, she discovered something, "I had more time. It is faster to pop one my meals into a microwave at a convenience store, or hospital cafeteria than actually stopping to buy food."

She was able to make more office visits and more sales calls than before. The cooler not only helped her change her physique in preparation for a contest, it made her life easier.

"I don't have to think about where I'm going to eat, what I'm going to eat. It is already with me in my cooler," she said.

Lynnie said the same thing, "While everyone else is rushing through their lunch break trying to eat, or rushing to get a snack on break. I don't have to rush and can actually take a break because my lunches are right here."

What seems like a daunting trade off at first—carrying around a cooler, eating only planned, often less flavorful foods—has an unforeseen benefit that reduces the cost of the trade-off to just the gastronomical aspect. And, as Lynnie says, "abs look better than anything tastes."

With that, I was ready to start working on the last piece of the puzzle.

I had the overload over time. Through tracking my lean muscle diameter and workout logs I had dialed in on my training. The Miami Muscle Girls taught me intensity. I knew the value of protein. It was time to make the trade-off and start tracking my diet.

—————— **CHAPTER SEVENTEEN** ——————
SUGAR IS THE ENEMY

"Are you sticking to the diet?" Lynn Suave, one of the Miami Muscle Girls asked me over the phone. "Yes," I replied.

"Are you doing your cardio?" she asked. "Yes," I said again.

We were all perplexed about what was happening.

I got stuck at 225 pounds. I was not losing body fat. My strength was holding steady. I was becoming just another version of that guy.

She pushed me some more, "are you really sticking to the diet?" "Yes!" I replied.

"Are you really doing your cardio?" she asked, her French accent growing thicker with frustration. "Yes, I am," I said. I was doing exactly what we had planned.

The Miami Muscle Girls' factory has churned out a lot of guys. In fact they train as many guys as girls. Even a few lower level professional male bodybuilders will consult with them for a back to basics tune up.

Lynn couldn't figure out why I got stuck so fast.

The quizzing went more in-depth. She asked me about my family, parents, siblings, aunts, uncles.

"Well, everyone in my family has been over weight," I told them.

"Ouffff, duh," Lynn said, her accent began relaxing now that she found the source of the problem. "Do you have a thermometer?"

That was the strangest question I had ever heard. I didn't have thermometer. She told me to go and get a digital one. Not the cheapest, not the most expensive. My new assignment—take my temperature every morning when I woke up.

The average body temperature for most people is somewhere around 98.6 degrees when they are awake and going about their daily tasks. During the day, my temperature is around 97.9 degrees. It has always run low.

In the morning, upon waking most people are somewhere at or just below 97.8 degrees. My average temperature upon waking is 97 degrees.

The daily temperature check showed that I had the symptoms of a thyroid problem. Knowing that I was running a bit cool is an indicator of a slow metabolism. I went to my doctor to determine two things:

1. What was my thyroid blood level
2. How well was my body metabolizing sugar and carbs

Only a doctor and lab work determine those two things with precision.

The thyroid screening is a simple blood test. Blood is drawn and sent to a lab.

The blood sugar insulin reaction is a little more involved. It is the glucose tolerance test used to diagnose diabetes. After fasting, blood is drawn. Then I drank a sugary solution and had blood drawn again, and then drank more of the sugary goo and had blood drawn again.

The tests showed what we were all thinking. I had a mild thyroid problem and terrible reaction to sugar. I didn't have diabetes, just a bad tolerance for sugar. My body didn't like to turn carbs and sugars into glycogen stored in the muscle for energy. It preferred to turn carbs into fat.

A lot of people who are overweight or have a hard time losing fat have the same double-whammy condition. It is actually rather common. My endocrinologist was surprised I didn't weight 300 pounds or more. All those years of workouts saved me from myself. If I hadn't been burning off so much energy with 'Armageddon Arm Workouts' I would have been seriously obese.

It would have been pretty easy, and perfectly reasonable, for me to say, "Hey, my body is fighting this fat loss thing too hard. I'll just have to be happy being a big heavy duty guy."

But, before I could get those words out of my mouth, Lynn said, "Oh, just like big Paul. Hmmm. You will just have to diet harder." And so I did.

Working counter-clockwise through my day, I gradually eliminated all sugars and carbs. The first carbs and sugars eliminated were the ones I ate in the evening. Then

I eliminated the carbs in the late afternoon. Like I said, I slowly eliminated all the carbs and sugars I ate going counter-clockwise, I eliminated the carbs I ate at 9 p.m., then eliminated the carbs I ate at 7 p.m.

It was a slow gradual process as we took advantage of the calorie and sugar deficit with each food eliminated. Once my body seemed to adapt to having fewer carbs and sugars, I eliminated some more.

But it was not all rainbows and flowers. I had to overcome one more addiction. And that addiction was at 2:30 p.m., 12:00 p.m. and 7:00 a.m. I was addicted to a meal replacement drink.

I loved that drink. It was smooth, sweet, thick. Just wonderful. But it was loaded with sugar and carbs.

I was still carrying some of the that guy mentality. That guy does stupid workouts. That guy doesn't track or measure anything. That guy thinks a supplement or meal replacement drink has some real magical potency.

The supplements are not magical. Notice how they come and go. For guys in your late 20s and 30s, think about all the supplements you have used. Think of how they were supposedly the silver bullet to build muscle and lose fat. They were advertised with top bodybuilders endorsing them, they were prominently featured at nutrition stores, then a year or so later they disappeared. They were replaced by something else. Something "better."

If one of them actually worked, it would have stuck around for more than a few years.

I had to get over my addiction to a meal replacement drink. I had to learn to eat real meals.

I resisted getting rid of the 2:30 p.m. addiction for more than a month. I was lying to myself. I told myself—"I need this, I need these carbs and sugars." Which was stupid because I knew from the blood tests I really didn't. I told myself, "Well, I guess this is as lean and light as I get." I didn't want to give up the sugar.

I finally dropped my 2:30 p.m. meal replacement drink. And guess what. I started getting a headache. Withdrawal. Predictable and treatable just like any headache with aspirin and acetaminophen. But then, my waist got smaller and I could see some more of my abs.

At this point I thought I had found my eating plan. I was slowly dropping pounds, I was maintaining my strength. Things were going great. For many people, cutting out the sugars and most of the carbs after their workout will be all they need to get pretty lean.

But there are some who want to get really lean. Maybe even something close to full-on ripped. And there are some people who are like me—who will hit a mega plateau.

If I wanted to keep getting leaner, I had to keep under loading the carbs and sugars. When I hit the plateau, I had to really under load. And the easiest target to eliminate is sugar.

Here's a look at my heavy duty diet in the hours leading up to my weight lifting.

- 6:00 a.m. Wake up

- Whey Protein Drink
    150 Cal
    27 g Protein
    2 g carbs

- Glutamine caps

- Cardio
    Run on treadmill @ 6.5 mph then walk 4 mph 1% incline

- 7:30 a.m. Meal Replacement Drink
    350 Cal
    32 g Protein
    12 g Carbs
    With a tablespoon of flax oil

- 9:45 a.m. 5 Jumbo eggs with cheese (5 whites, 1 Yolk) and 14 g cheese
    155 Cal
    30.5 g Protein
    3 g carbs

- 11:00 a.m. Chicken meal
    - 150 g of charcoal grilled chicken breast
    - 75 g sweet potato
    - 35 g broccoli
    - 14 g cheese

    - 390 Calories
    - 45 g protein
    - 16.75 g carbs

- 12:00 noon Meal Replacement Drink
    - 350 cal
    - 32 g protein
    - 12 g carbs

- 1:00 Lift weights M, W, F Run sprints, plymetrics, agility T, Th

The obvious thing to replace here is my old nemesis, the meal replacement drink. It has sugar in it. The meal replacement drink became 150 grams of steak and 75 grams of sweet potato. Eventually, even all the sweet potato would go away.

Before I got started down the drastic no-carb path, I eliminated the sugars in a steady, systematic way, moving counter-clockwise through the day. Which made the logical and obvious target from my heavy duty eating plan the 12:00 p.m. meal replacement drink.

But I had another addiction. The substitution of the meal replacement drink with steak brought out that addiction.

Moving backward through the day, a counter-clockwise elimination of carbs and sugars is the easiest way to lose fat. Eliminating carbs and sugars before you go to bed is an easy first step, then, eliminate all the sugars and carbs from earlier in the evening. Gradually, move counter clockwise through the day eliminating carbs and sugars and you will be amazed at the results from something so simple. Except it really isn't so simple. Sugar is highly addictive.

Researchers from Princeton recently presented a study to the American College of Neuropsychopharmacology showing that sugar exhibits the same addictive patterns as cocaine. Sugar, especially a binge, releases dopamine, just like other drugs.

When the dopamine is burned off there is the withdrawal and craving. It is not just the taste of the cupcake that is so tempting, the neuro-chemical reaction that feels so good is a large part of the equation.

I recommend cutting the sugars slowly, counter clockwise, starting at the end of the day because it is the easiest way to beat the withdrawal and wean a person off the addiction. If a person can beat the addiction to sugar and then carbs, it may bring out another addiction in most people. An addiction that can derail a plan to lose fat.

If you have to be addicted to anything, being addicted to being strong is a pretty damn good thing to be addicted to.

When I cut out my 12:00 p.m. meal replacement drink, my strength decreased. I went into a stupid panic, "I can only do dumbbell bench press with 100 pounders for six reps!" The horror!

I was about ready to pull the plug on this fat loss project. My weight was down. I was leaner, lighter. But I did not want to give up my strength. My strength was part of my identity. I was a big, strong, heavy duty guy who could move a lot of weight. Now I was becoming a smaller not so strong guy.

I didn't want to go back to being that guy. He always does lifts that are really easy to move heavy poundages on. Everyone can do a crappy set of toerisers with a couple hundred pounds. Everyone can do a crappy set of shrugs with 315 pounds. That guy lets his identity get caught up with an amount of weight.

He also does bench on the smith machine with 405 pounds, which is actually 360 pounds for one or two reps, taking a five minute rest between sets and guzzling a sports drink. Is he accomplishing much? Not really. But it makes him feel good. It helps his ego. It gives him an identity.

I was confronted with the question, who did I want to be.

The Miami Muscle Girls talked me into sticking with it for two more weeks.

Two weeks later I was down to 217 pounds. My top two abs were fully visible and I could start to see a four pack.

I decided I wanted to be a lean muscular guy.

The next move was easier. I got rid of cheese. This brought down my total caloric intake without any real effect on strength or muscle and no withdrawal. It also brought my waist down even more and separation started to show up between my delts/triceps/biceps.

Now I was hooked.

I finally kicked the 7:00 a.m. meal replacement addiction. Bye-bye sugary drink, hello oatmeal. One big cup of oatmeal, with a scoop of whey protein, flax oil, cinnamon and Splenda. And when I say one big cup, I actually mean 80 grams of oatmeal. Everything is measured to the gram.

That was an amazing change. I was actually taking in more carbs, but my sugars went down to 12 grams.

My loss of strength—which can correlate to a loss of muscle—stabilized.

Substituting some the expensive, fancy, hi-tech meal replacement drink for old fashioned oatmeal was a huge change. Veins came out in my biceps. The 4-pack became more pronounced, the fat on my lower pecs melted away.

NITA SPEAKS _____

Identity, a person's **self image**, is one the most powerful forces in the universe. We build it and protect it. We will avoid risks that might damage it. The tragedy is in when we let our identity get in the way of **our dreams and goals**.

When we cling so hard to our established self image that we don't **let ourselves grow and improve**. We then talk ourselves out of our goals and dreams. We become the biggest obstacle to our own happiness.

The only solution is to accept what a powerful force self image is and **focus on the dream** and the goal which in turn will create new self image.

I held steady on this system of two carb meals for two months. I actually started to get a bit stronger.

The morning runs got longer. Then 20 minutes walking on the treadmill before I lifted weights, grew to 40 minutes.

At this point, my weight lifting regime had changed, but the tracking stayed and so did the overload over time.

The principles of over load are immutable—even when fighting a defensive battle to hold onto muscle while trying to lose fat.

Twelve weeks later, I was down to 210 pounds. My only carbs came from a cup of oatmeal after my morning cardio.

Three weeks later, I was down to a third of a cup of oatmeal as my only intentional carbs for the whole day!

That sucked.

But, the reflection in the mirror was looking better. I was losing strength and by 2:00 p.m. and I really couldn't concentrate on much. Luckily, I front loaded all my work into the early morning.

After 15 weeks I was down to 202 pounds.

The Miami Muscle Girls asked if I wanted to take one last step. The step that separates competitive bodybuilders from the merely serious enthusiast: Ketosis.

Ketosis is the crucible. For the Miami Muscle Girls, it determines whether they will keep you as serious training client. And getting the fat off is a serious test.

Ketosis is when your body, deprived of all carbs and sugars, converts fat to ketones to be used as energy. It is the principle behind the Atkins diet and the South Beach diet. But these girls take it to a whole new level.

I had to go to the drug store to buy Keto Strips. They are used to detect the ketones in the urine to determine if my body was producing ketones. It is easy to screw up a ketogenic diet by eating just a few carbs (the precise application of ketogenic diet is detailed in Part II of this book).

Normally a bodybuilder on a contest diet only goes Ketogenic at the very end, to go from ripped to shredded.

I needed to be ketogenic to from soft to relatively lean. I survived three of their 12 day cycles and got down to 193 pounds.
Honestly, I looked like shit—kinda lean, stringy, flat.

Then I went back up to a full cup of oatmeal for breakfast. Whomp! Within a week I was at 198 pounds and my muscles looked full and round.

We had found my "base" diet. Even now, it is still pretty close to what I've listed below.

- Pre-Breakfast - Whey protein with water
- Cardio
- Meal #1 - 1 Cup oatmeal, whey protein, Flax Oil
- Meal #2 - 6 egg whites, two yolks
- Meal #3 - Steak, veggies
- Lift weights
- Meal #4 - Whey protein with water
- Meal #5 - 6 Egg whites, two yolks
- Meal #6 Steak or Talapia, veggies
- Meal #7 - Steak or Talapia, veggies
- Meal #8 - Whey Protein with water

If you notice, **this eating plan is comprised of basic foods**. No exotic drinks or supplements. No potions that claim they will volumize the cells.

During this whole process I never took any fat burners—no clenbuterol, ephedra or anything else.

My supplementation is very pedestrian—glutamine, amino acid tabs, multi vitamin, B6, B12, calcium and whey protein.

The full description of the ketogenic carb cycles I used then and still use are in Part II. The cycles are pretty straight forward, but also really easy to get wrong.

They are tough, but they work, they can actually become kind of addictive. But they should only be used when nothing else breaks the plateau.

I was where I wanted to be in terms of weight and leanness. My strength came back. But I was still missing one last piece of the puzzle for being truly 'Fit for Combat' and a training and diet regime to maintain it.

The remaining item was my cardio training.

CHAPTER EIGHTEEN
COMBAT CARDIO

"Hey sir, are we running?" the soldier yelled.

A second later I was sprinting along with Captain Robby Johnson and PFC Randolph Kloos down a street in Baghdad toward a known terrorist leader.

Johnson and Kloos had their guns up, I had my TV camera on my shoulder.

In the maze of buildings and passage ways that make up urban Baghdad, foot speed is essential. A gunman can slip into corridor, inside a house then squirt out the back courtyard. The soldiers train to build their burst speed and my sprinting work allowed me to keep up with them.

We closed the distance fast and rounded a corner. The soldiers had him. Then machine gun fire echoed off the walls and buildings.

It was a typical day in Baghdad.

The bodybuilders who just flex on stage don't run. But I'm not a bodybuilder. I work in a war zone and being able to run is a must. But there is another category of bodybuilder who does run.

At this stage in my goal to become truly 'Fit for Combat', I was running a lot and starting to resemble a bodybuilder. The bodybuilders who run, have a lot of muscle, and are really lean with Olympic level stamina and power are women's fitness competitors.

They run. They run a lot. They do distance, sprints, middle-distance, plyometrics anything that will get their heart to the bursting point.

If these women can carry extraordinary amounts of muscle around, while running and with the power and stamina to do their routines—they are worth listening to. Nita Marquez is one of them and I listened to her.

What I learned from her is that I was doing my running all wrong. I was thinking about my cardio conditioning the wrong way.

Just about every fitness center has some serious runners as members. These people log 20 to 40 miles a week and are in great cardio vascular condition—but most of them look remarkably average. They do not have much muscle and many of them are skinny fat.

The best explanation for this phenomena came from my friend Lisa Krog. Lisa and her husband Glen are the top trainers in Johannesburg, South Africa. Like Lynn Suave and the Miami Muscle Girls, they have a factory churning out physique competitors. Lisa and Glen explained cardio to me like this:

> "If the energy in, energy out formula worked, you would be able to cardio yourself out of existence.

> If you did enough cardio every day to burn 500 more calories than you ate, after a few years you would simply not exist. But all those people putting in hours on the cardio machines for years still exist."

That was an odd way to put it, but it does show the flaw in the energy in, energy out formula.

It is really hard to exercise and cardio the fat off because the body will adapt. Lisa and Glenn also explained the effects of long term cardio like running on the body:

> "Firstly cardiovascular activity is very efficient at chewing up muscle tissue, the steps are as follows:

> 1. Conversion from fast twitch muscle fiber to slow twitch muscle fiber, by acquiring mitochondria and relinquishing contractile protein. Smaller fiber, lower resting metabolic rate and fewer calories burned when not exercising.

> 2. Excessive Cortisol released in response to the damage to the fiber as a result of the exercise. Cortisol acts as a natural analgesic, but severely hampers protein synthesis and muscle repair. It also damages the immune system, and ultimately will contribute to all of our deaths - so I'm not sure why anyone would do anything that would accelerate this process.

> 3. It has been shown, that high volume cardiovascular exercise can completely deplete satellite cells in muscle fiber, which means no new

fiber can grow or existing fiber be repaired.

4. Growth Hormone levels decline with high volume cardiovascular exercise, which also hampers the repair process. Low growth hormone also accelerates aging.

5. To sum it up, you can't train all day, and you can't eat no food, but you can always build a bit more muscle, so quit the cardio and concentrate on the weight lifting."

That was a very strong argument for not doing cardio. But I need to be able to keep up with Paratroopers and U.S. Marines in combat. Cardio conditioning is a must for me. And, I need strength and power.

The solution was to train like an International Federation of Bodybuilding professional female fitness athlete—specifically, one that always wins the fitness routine portion of the contest. In other words, I needed to start training like Nita.

And what does she do? Sprints.

Nita and Lisa flipped the cardio equation on me.

If all I cared about was my physical appearance, Lisa would advise that I do zero cardio. Nita, being a fitness competitor, has to have the physical appearance and the stamina/power to do her fitness routine at contests.

The best way to gain cardio conditioning and maintain muscle is to do what Nita does—sprints.

I was always doing some sprints, but I treated them as 'functional' training and distance running as my cardio conditioning. Nita, a petite IFBB professional fitness athlete, flipped that idea on its head.

Sprinting became the core of my cardio conditioning program and distance running became the 'functional' training.

When I started doing sprints in the morning for my cardio, my strength gains in the gym accelerated, I started to get leaner without really trying and the lean muscle diameter of my upper arm started improving.

Now I was truly 'Fit for Combat'. I was light at 204 pounds, was stronger than I would ever need to be in Iraq or Afghanistan, had burst speed and explosiveness, and I had the stamina and endurance to keep up with anyone.

The cardio was the last element of what I now think of as a system. A system that a few people have started to adopt. After I came back from my most recent trip to Iraq, where I gained a few pounds of fat and lost a few pounds of muscle, I ran through the system again. People started to notice at the gym and began asking me questions.

A few took exactly what I said and started doing it. And it worked.

The system (which will be explained in full detail in Part II) works not because it is a one sized fits all program. It works because it is a systematic way for a person to find what works for them by going back to the fundamentals and working it through step by step. In that regard, the system is a rational approach to solving a problem.

The only time the system breaks down is when a person behaves like a human—irrationally.

NITA SPEAKS

With high-intensity interval training you "sprint" on any cardio exercise for short bursts that go for less than two minutes, and then you slow it down to moderate, and sometimes even low-intensity pace for a short burst. You want to go high intensity to kick your heart rate way up, and then you drop the intensity to let your body rest, while not giving your heart rate enough time to drop out beneath a fat-burning zone. If you do this for short bursts of time, you don't give your heart rate a chance to drop severely, and therein, you are able to keep your body burning fat, burning calories, and staying hard at work, even though you won't feel like you're working hard while your body recovers during your lower-paced durations.

Like cardio, this too can strengthen your heart, and keep you from feeling sluggish. On the other hand, in comparison to cardio, interval training burns fat for longer periods of time. You will burn fat for up to 13 hours post-workout with intervals, whereas with cardio at a constant moderate rate will only burn fat efficiently for up to 2 hours post-workout. So, why would you spend more time and burn less fat, much less want to gamble the possibility of kicking out cortisol? This is why many fitness professionals who know what they are doing will not recommend long, boring, high, low or medium-intensity periods of cardio.

CHAPTER NINETEEN
IRRATIONALLY HUMAN

Humans are hard wired to avoid loss. Humans find comfort in the familiar.

When we lose something we value, or face the potential of losing something we value, we experience psychological pain in the form of anxiety.

We don't like to change. I didn't want to change what I was doing in the gym.

In the 'Fit for Combat' system you will encounter this a lot. You will be forced to give things up. You may lose some of your favorite exercises which were so fun because they you were so good at them.

In a few pages you will go through Phase I. If you follow it, you will lose a lot of the old familiar workouts you used to do. You will resist it. When people commit to an idea, it is hard to turn away from it. Back when I was that guy I was committed to a lot of weird workout ideas—like having to do a lot of exercises. I was committed to the idea that if I wasn't sore the next day, I didn't workout hard enough.

Muscle soreness is not a measurement of progress. And the number of exercises you do doesn't matter. But it is hard to give those things up.

In Phase II, you will lose a lot of fat, but you may also lose strength and muscle size, which is why the Miami Muscle Girls use the diet as the true test of commitment.

In Phase III and beyond, you may lose some of the definition you achieved in Phase II, but will be able to maintain a lean muscular physique and know the tools to always gradually improve your physique.

Dan Ariely, a business professor at the Massachusetts Institute of Technology, says humans are predictably irrational. We humans become even more irrational in our decision making when faced with the loss of something we value.

For me it was hard to give up dips. I valued dips even though they were completely useless to me. I did not value the benefit of doing dips because the benefit ceased years before when I was never able to increase the number of reps or weight. But I still did them. Why?

I valued how cool it looked to be able to do dips with three 45 pound plates chained around my waist.

I kept telling myself I wanted to build muscle, and lose fat. But what I really valued was the comfort, the self-esteem and self-identity derived from being the guy who could do dips with three 45 pound plates chained around his waist.

My actions did not match my stated goals. I was being irrational. Irrational behavior is completely predictable in humans.

When I tell you to change your workout, you will have to give things up. Some of you will not follow one word of the advise in this book because it advises you to change what you are doing. And you will not want to lose the familiarity of what you are doing. You have committed to something and it is hard to break that. Even if it is horribly irrational and producing no results.

But, if what you were doing was really working, would you have bought this book? Is what you are doing now really working?

The changes from what you are doing now to Phase I will cause some anxiety. There will be a sense of loss. But you can get through it.

We all value muscle. We've worked too damned hard to get it to lose it. When confronted with anything that would cause us to lose muscle or strength, we will resist it.

For those who follow through on Phase II, the fat loss may become addictive. If a person is focused on being lean, they will never move back to building up muscle in Phase III. We all value being lean but, you will have to give a little of that up to build muscle.

When I explain to people what I do to look and perform the way I do, they often hesitate. Many people are reluctant about keeping a training log—even if they do not change their workout! Just the idea of keeping track of their lifts causes discomfort.

If you have been working out for years you will probably continue to work out for years. What then, I ask, is the loss of keeping a log book? There is none, but it is change. It is not what you have been doing and that is a loss.

An extreme example of this was portrayed by Ori & Rom Brafman in their book, Sway.

The Brafman's relate the story of the founder of a bio-tech company that went public on the stock exchange. The founder the company saw the stock price rise and become a multi-millionaire overnight. His investment advisor told him to cash in, sell the stock, and diversify. The founder decided to hold on to his stock. As the tech-bubble burst, he started chasing the loss. He was convinced that the stock would get back up to its previous high. He thought selling at any price below the high was a loss. Rather than cash out and still make a million bucks, he held on to his stock. He refused to take the imagined loss. And they key is imagined. If he would have sold, it would have been a net gain. But he compared the sale at $20 per share to the high of $50 per share to a $30 loss.

In the end, as the Brafman's describe it, the stock wound up only worth a few dollars a share.

The founder of the company had chased the loss all the way down to a $48 dollar loss.

For people like me, who are experimenters, or as the marketers call us, 'early adopters', trying a new workout, even a useless one, is in our DNA.

But for most people, trying something new is daunting. Some people may be so afraid of losing what they have, they will not change. They see where they are as being at the top, and anything—anything—that could change it, could cause a loss.

But you really don't have anything to lose by keeping a log book and overloading over time.

You will lose the same thing I had to lose when I started down this path—my pride in that I knew what I was doing.

I thought I was a really smart workout guy back then. I realize now I didn't know much.

Before I started really analyzing my workouts and tracking my progress, I valued those crazy workouts. I cobbled them together—a little bit of 'Armageddon Arm Workout' a little bit of something else—viola, I'm a workout genius! I would experiment with anything—as long as I felt like I owned it.

To admit that they did not work, was to admit that I didn't really know a whole a lot about what I was doing. Pride. And losing your pride is a very tough thing.

When I admitted to myself what I was doing wasn't working, that I was not making progress, that's when changes started to occur. I started doing Coach Rosenfield workouts. I found the best training advice from women bodybuilders. The best diet advice from a bikini contest winner. And the best cardio program from a 4'9" fitness competitor.

And I'm proud to have done it all. Because bottom line, it works.

What follows from here is a step-by-step explanation of the 'Fit for Combat' system. It works every time on every body because it follows a few immutable physiological laws—like overload over time leading to muscle hypertrophy over time.

The open architecture of the system is deliberate. Every person is different which is why I use quantifiable measurements like lean muscle diameter. This system, if followed, will lead you to the diet and weight lifting program that works for you. All you have to do is quit being irrational.

So, lets get started.

— PART II —

FIT FOR COMBAT SYSTEMS

CHAPTER TWENTY
PHASE I

Phase I, Step One: Build the Muscle

There are a couple good reasons to build the muscle first. For starters, building muscle is the least complicated part of this system. Second, it is the easiest. Third, it yields the most tangible results. Fourth, it is the most fun.

Finally, (this is the main reason) building the muscle first is what worked for me and countless others.

Muscle is the foundation of this system. The amount of muscle you carry plays a large role in your metabolic rate. It determines the shape of your body. Muscle gives you speed and power.

For me, in the beginning stage, every exercise built muscle. Muscle equals strength and power. In this phase it is best to concentrate on the basics, getting the maximum out of every set.

When you are getting the maximum out of every set, you do not need to do a bunch of sets or a bunch of exercises. The body responds to overload. So you need to overload the muscle every set. And spread that overload over time.

NITA SPEAKS

A lot of my clients when they first come to me are shocked when I tell them "you don't have an excess body fat problem, you have a lack of muscle problem." Even people who have been working out for years can have a lack of muscle problem.

Muscle burns calories. The more muscle you have, the easier it is to lose fat. Therefore, Phase I, building more muscle, comes first.

Building muscle is the triple threat of fat loss. You burn calories during the weight lifting. You burn calories as your body recovers from the weight lifting (hypertrophy!). And, after the hypertrophy, the increased muscle mass burns more calories even while you are being a lazy ass watching TV!

The other reason you need to build the muscle first is if you go just go into diet and fat loss, you will wind up being scrawny and lean or even worse—skinny fat

In starting out Phase I, you want to keep it very simple. Make it very results oriented. So simple, in fact, you are not even going to use barbells or dumbbells. A couple people are probably rolling their eyes right now saying to themselves, "But JD, big barbells build big muscles."

Yes they do. But machines have a great advantage in the beginning of Phase I. They allow you to focus on only moving heavier and heavier poundages without having to worry about form or technique.

Bench pressing 225 pounds with a barbell requires a lot of athletic coordination. Bench pressing 70 pound dumbbells requires even more athletic coordination. Moving 240 pounds on a machine chest press just requires muscle. With a machine you are able to concentrate on putting all your energy into moving the stack of weight rather than balancing the weight.

And again our goal here in the beginnings of Phase I is to build the damn muscle.

To start out with our machine centered beginnings of Phase I, here is a pretty good workout:.

Workout #1
- CHEST PRESS MACHINE (Any kind)
- SHOULDER PRESS MACHINE (Any kind)
- TRICEP PUSH DOWNS (Straight or slightly angled bar)

Two sets of each exercise. Pick a number, any number between 12 and 16. That number is now your Magic Number. Your goal is to get that many reps over the course of two sets. Here is how I keep track of it in my training log:

Seated Chest Press
285 x 7
     x 4
Total 11

My magic number for the beginning of Phase I is 15. And here is the key. **YOU MUST STICK WITH YOUR MAGIC NUMBER.** It does not matter what your number is **BUT YOU MUST STICK WITH YOUR MAGIC NUMBER.**

So, in this example my total reps were 11. My Magic Number is 15. So, the next time I do Workout #1, I have to beat 11 reps.

So, lets follow this over the course of a few weeks.

>*Week 1*
>Seated Chest Press
>285 x 7
>   x 5
>Total 12
>
>*Week 2*
>Seated Chest Press
>285 x 10
>   x 5
>Total 15
>
>*Week 3*
>Seated Chest Press
>295 x 6
>   x 4
>Total 10
>
>*Week 4*
>Seated Chest Press
>295 x 8
>   x 4
>Total 12
>
>*Week 5*
>Seated Chest Press
>295 x 11
>   x 6
>Total 17
>
>*Week 6*
>305 x 5
>   x 3
>Total 8

See the pattern? Pretty straight forward. This is what I mean by overload over time.

The muscle is constantly being forced to do more work either through increased reps or increased weight.

Now, what happens if you can't go up in reps.

> *Week 6*
> Seated Chest Press
> 305 x 5
>   x 3
> Total 8

Did you have an off day? Did you get all your meals in? Did you get enough sleep? Did you go to the dentist before lifting weights?

A lot of variables can come into play. So, try it again.

> *Week 7*
> Seated Chest Press
> 305 x 5
>   x 3
> Total 8

At this point I call the Seated Chest Press, DONE! No need to waste any more gym time doing the same weight, for the same reps. Doing the same weight for the same reps is the opposite of overload over time. Hell, it is the opposite of overload. It is just plain stupid. And as I mentioned before, I spent a lot of time being just plain stupid. So, no more of that.

Eventually, one of two things will happen. You will not be able to increase reps or weight. Or, on the machines you will run out of weight. How many of you have actually gotten to the point where you have outgrown a machine? Using this system, some of you will. And that is one of the coolest feelings in the world. Which is why we start off with building strength and muscle in Phase I.

But if either of those two things happens—no big deal. That just gives us an opportunity to move on to something new. A new machine to outgrow.

Once you outgrow the Seated Chest Press, or as illustrated above, plateau, try a machine incline press.

But here is the twist. Make Machine Incline Press your last exercise of Workout #1. Here's a refresher of the original Workout #1.

> *Workout #1*
> • CHEST PRESS MACHINE (Any kind)
> • SHOULDER PRESS MACHINE (Any kind)
> • TRICEP PUSH DOWNS (Straight or slightly angled bar)

After you have worn out chest press machine, by outgrowing the machine or because you can no longer increase the weight or reps and have called it DONE, you need to change the exercise. Instead of putting the new chest exercise in the same order, move it to the end of the workout, like below:

> *Workout #1*
> • SHOULDER PRESS MACHINE (Any kind)
> • TRICEP PUSH DOWNS (Straight or slightly angled bar)
> • MACHINE INCLINE PRESS (Any kind)

This ensures accuracy of tracking.

If your tracking is off, how do you know if you are really making progress overloading your muscles over time? Throwing a brand new exercise in front of an exercise will throw off your tracking a lot. But moving an exercise to last in your workout is less disruptive. And if you are in the new order, you will be able to keep moving up in weight and reps with shoulder press. So, the only time you change the order of your exercises is when you change up after maxing on an exercise.

Let me reiterate this. **DON'T CHANGE THE ORDER OF YOUR EXERCISES**. Once you settle on a workout, don't change the order, it will throw off your tracking.

Now think about this for a second. How often have you seen workouts listed somewhere as three sets of ten reps.

As in doing three sets of shoulder press for ten reps on each set.

If ten reps was your failure point on the first set, then on the next set you will only be able to do six reps and probably only four reps on the third set. The only way to keep getting the prescribed ten reps is to reduce the weight.

Or, even worse, a person thinks there is some mystical muscle magic in three sets of ten reps. So they pick a weight that will allow them to get ten reps every set, at which point they are really only working to failure on the last set—if at all.

If you are not taking a set to failure, you are not really overloading the muscle. And that is the mistake I made for a long time.

The muscle only responds to overload, by increasing the stress. To make that muscle grow you have to overload it. There are four things that can happen when you overload the muscle on a given repetition:

1. You complete the repetition
2. You only kind of move the weight
3. You don't move the weight at all
4. You tear the muscle

Luckily #4 is very rare, #1, #2 and #3 lead to muscle growth. The goal is to get to that overload and increase that overload every workout.

The most straightforward way to do that is how I illustrated it above. Basic exercises taking every set to failure. Increase the rep load until a goal number of reps is achieved then increasing the weight. Keep track of the time between sets by using a clock on the wall, stop watch or counting breaths. One minute or less between sets is a good starting point for Step One.

When you cannot increase the weight or reps, move on to another exercise that works the same muscle groups.

At this point you also need to start keeping track of the lean muscle diameter of your upper arm. Back in Chapter 3, I explained how I used a cloth tape measure, body fat calipers and the mathematical constant of Pi (3.14) to track whether I was actually building muscle. (Lean muscle diameter will be explained in more detail in Chapter 21.) You will want to keep track of lean muscle diameter because that is how you will know for certain if these workouts are working for you and how to gauge the adjustments made through all the phases. Lean muscle diameter is how you find the workout that works best for you.

Now, lets look at the basic Phase I, Step One workout we will start with.

As I mentioned before, I was addicted to dips. You may be addicted to an exercise as well. If you are not sure, it's the exercises you do faithfully even though they have long since ceased to work. I had to throw dips away. You may have to overcome some of those irrational addictions as well.

There are probably three or maybe four really effective workouts for building up muscle and power in Step One. At the beginnings of Step One, machines are our best friends.

Lets take Workout #1 listed above.

> *Workout #1*
> • CHEST PRESS MACHINE (Any kind)
> • SHOULDER PRESS MACHINE (Any kind)
> • TRICEP PUSH DOWNS (Straight or slightly angled bar)

Do this workout on Monday, Sunday, or Tuesday. The exact day does not matter because we will call whatever day you start as day one. And since there are only seven days in the week, the numbers here are really small.

> **Day One**
> *Workout #1*
> • CHEST PRESS MACHINE (Any kind)
> • SHOULDER PRESS MACHINE (Any kind)
> • TRICEP PUSH DOWNS (Straight or slightly angled bar)
>
> **Day Two**
> • Off or Short Duration Sprints
>
> **Day Three**
> *Workout #2*
> • LEG PRESS
> • LEG CURLS
> • CALVES (any exercise)
>
> **Day Four**
> • Off
>
> **Day Five**
> *Workout # 3*
> • LAT PULLDOWNS (any grip)

• BARBELL CURLS (straight or EZ)
• SHRUGS (Any kind)

Day Six
• Off or Short Duration Sprints

Day Seven
• Off

You will want to start off doing only two sets of each exercise to failure. The reason for doing such low volume is to help you find the workout that works best for you. I do not know your genetic capacity for hypertrophy or how fast you can recover from a workout, so it is better to start out with a low-volume, low frequency, higher intensity program and then increase the volume and frequency.

As you track your progress in your log book and lean muscle diameter, you will be able to quantify the gains and the results of each adjustment to determine if it works for you.

If you are addicted any of the exercises above—and we all know how bad being addicted to an exercise can be—substitute another.

How long does step one last? Ah…now, normally you would expect someone to say four weeks, or two months. Right? But what does four weeks or two months have to do with overload over time?

Nothing.

A measurement like days, weeks or months is arbitrary. Think about what we track in the log books. Progress. Increases in weight and reps. Increases in lean muscle diameter.

How will you know if you have made enough progress to move to step two?

How many exercises have you plateaued on? How much has your lean muscle diameter increased?

There are nine exercises in step one. Two of them are tough to plateau on—Leg Press and Shrugs. Most guys, even *that guy,* can shrug and leg press a lot. So there are seven likely plateau exercises. When you have plateaued and substituted four exercises you are probably ready for step two of Phase I. If your lean muscle diameter has improved, but the rate of increase is slowing down or stopped, it is probably time to make an adjustment to step two.

It may take you a few weeks, for some guys it will take months. But what you will find is that you are able to become stronger than you thought and as long as you are making progress in step one, there is no reason to change things up.

The principles of step one of Phase I are simple. Machines allow you to concentrate on building strength and muscle, tracking and consistency. It is all about getting you into the habit of tracking, overloading over time and holding yourself accountable.

Now some of you may have noticed something. I suggest barbell curls instead of some type of machine curl. Easy answer. Most gyms don't have a decent machine that works the biceps. A lot of gyms have bicep machines that are awkward contraptions. But, if your gym has a straight forward preacher curls machine, use that instead of barbell curls.

And of course there is the elephant in the room that is not mentioned as part of step one, Phase I, diet. I am tempted to say don't worry about it, just keep eating the way you are eating but I know there are some guys who are not eating enough protein. So, here is your step one diet plan. Eat whatever you want just get one gram of protein in you per pound of body weight.

Jump on a scale. How much do you weigh? Okay, eat that many grams of protein. Steak, fish, chicken, eggs, pork, soy, whey, whatever.

For example, if you weigh 210 pounds, take in 210 grams of protein. If you weigh 170 pounds, take in 170 grams of protein. And protein is the priority nutrient. When you eat a meal, eat all your protein sources first. No bread, no pasta, nothing until you have finished your protein source.

Protein is the priority food group from here on out.

For the ladies, protein intake can be tough. Many women do not digest protein as well as men and usually have problems digesting steak and chicken. Whey protein and eggs tend to be easier for women to digest. In this stage, women should try to get .6 grams of protein per pound of body weight. If a woman weighs 130 pounds, she should try to eat 78 grams of protein.

Simple enough? Good. So, after you have plateaued out on four exercises, and/or if your gains in lean muscle diameter have stopped or are slowing down, move on to step two.

Phase I, Step Two: Volume and Frequency

Now that you have been using the principle of overload overtime, you should start to see come changes. Works pretty good, eh?

Wait until you get into step two.

The principles of the weight training remain the same. Overload overtime, tracking, basic lifts, every set to failure.

In Step Two of Phase I we are going to change some things. There are three basic components to a workout program, volume, intensity and frequency. Volume being the number of exercises and sets, intensity being how hard you work and frequency being how often you work a given a muscle.

In step one, I had you start of with the old reliable--three exercises three times a week program. The volume was low, the intensity was high and the frequency was every seven days. The goal here in step two is to start finding the volume, intensity and frequency that work best for you. And we are going to do it gradually.

Often, people make wild swings in their workout programs. They may have been doing a low volume, high intensity program and then when the gains slow down or stop, they go to the opposite end of the spectrum with some insane high volume workout. A more precise course of action would be to make minor adjustments which allow for more precise tracking.

I'm going to give you two options. Option A, you increase the volume. Option B, you increase the frequency.

In Option A, you stick with the old reliable program from step one, but add one more set to failure. Instead of doing two sets of each exercise, add a third set.

In Option B, things get shook up a little bit more as the frequency is increased. Here's an Option B workout:

> *Workout #1*
> • Barbell or Dumbbell Bench Press
> • Barbell or Dumbbell Shoulder Press
> • Barbell Rows or Power Pulls
> • Wide Grip Skull Crushers or Bench Dips

• Shrugs of any kind

Workout #2
• Barbell or Dumbbell curls
• Squats or Any kind of leg press
• Leg Curls of any kind
• Toe risers of any kind

That's it. Almost too easy. You will still want to do only two sets to failure, because what is being adjusted is the frequency the muscles are hit.

The workout order illustrated below becomes mind numbingly repetitive. Again, it doesn't matter whether you start on Sunday or Tuesday because there are seven days in a week and we like to keep it simple.

Day One
Workout #1

Day Two
Off or Short Duration Sprints

Day Three
Workout #2

Day Four
Off

Day Five
Workout #1

Day Six
Off or Short Duration Sprints

Day Seven
Off

Day One
Workout #2

Day Two
Off

Day Three
Workout #1

Day Four
Off or Short Duration Sprints

Day Five
Workout #2

See the pattern. Pretty simple. Just rotate Workout #1 and Workout #2 and do not do sprints the day after Workout #2. Let your legs recover and soak up nutrients.

The substitution principle still applies and always will. When you plateau on an exercise, find a new one that works the same muscle group. Machines are still good, but try to find more barbell dumbbell moves. Think big lifts.

Option B adds another element to overload overtime—frequency of overload. But, you still need time to repair so the muscle can soak up protein and nutrients to rebuild itself. This rotation strikes a great balance between frequency and recovery time.

The muscle grows when it is stressed, when it is overloaded. The more frequently you can overload the muscle the more times it will be forced to grow.

Option A adds greater volume, a little more overload and micro-trauma to be recovered from.

Will it work for you? That is what we will find out. That is what we are testing.

By tracking your workouts in your log book and keeping track of your lean tissue diameter, you will be able to tell after a few months if the changes worked for you.

What we are looking for here is velocity in improvement or overall plateau. If you have been steadily making gains during step one, these changes may increase the velocity of the gains. If the velocity of strength and lean tissue gains picks up, this adjustment is getting you closer to your optimal hyper-trophy zone. If the velocity decreases or gains stop, then we have a couple options.

If you picked Option B and your velocity has stopped, we've learned a little bit about your recovery time. You may not be able to recover properly in three or five days, which is an important thing to know. Some people need up to 14 days to fully recover. A person who needs 14 days to recover, but is hitting a muscle every five days is going to be really frustrated.

So, if Option B is not working, try Option A.

If you picked Option A and your gains have slowed down or come to a complete halt we've learned about how much overload and micro-trama your body can recover from in six days. Adding more frequency will probably have the same effect. So, what can be adjusted? Volume, frequency and intensity can be adjusted.

This is Option C, which is actually the entire crux of this book and is fully explained in Chapter 21.

If Option A didn't work, pick something, volume, frequency, intensity. Just pick one so all the other variables can be controlled. Have you picked one? Good. Okay, if you picked volume, go back to the original old reliable from step one.

If you picked frequency, add in another day off from training. A day where you don't lift or run sprints. Take three days off between Workout #3 and Workout #1. Or, take two days off between Workout #2 and Workout #3. There is no law that says when you have to take days off or how many in a row. The bodybuilding police will not come and arrest you. What you do have to do is find the amount of time it takes for you to recover enough so you can continue to make gains.

If you picked intensity, just do two failure sets or one failure set. Treat the other set or two as warm up's and only take one set to extreme muscle crushing failure. For example, if you were doing chest press with 250 pounds you would start of with a warm up set of say 180 pounds for a few reps, then another set with say 230 pounds for a few reps then do your real set with 250 pounds to absolute failure. For tracking purposes, the failure set is what really counts. Just try to keep the warm up sets consistent.

What I've done in the preceding paragraphs is lay out the most important aspect of this program—finding what works for you! Using quantifiable measurements, tracking and minor adjustments to find the work out program that works best for you, is the only way to be successful in the gym over the long and even short haul. It really never ends. The longer you workout, the more dialed in you will get and the more your body will adapt and even optimize to where you will need to continue to make gradual adjustments to maintain progress.

You may have noticed something else—we never work our abs. The reason is if you are lifting hard, you are working your abs on every rep. And what your abs look like is not determined by exercise but diet. But if you really want to work your abs, throw in a set or two once a week.

On the topic of diet, you should be up to the grams of protein per pound of body weight I suggested in step one. You may have found that to get 170 grams of protein or 210 grams you had to substitute a lot of crap for meat, eggs, whey, soy, etc.

A few of you probably chucked some of the sugar and carbs aside when protein became the priority food group and you probably lost a few pounds of fat. Whoa, gaining muscle, getting stronger and losing fat!

In step two we will increase the protein a little to 1.25 grams of protein for every pound of body weight for the guys.

If you weigh 170 pounds you will eat 212 grams of protein [170 x 1.25=212]. If you weigh 210 pounds you will eat 262 grams of protein [210 x 1.25 = 262].

For women, try getting up to .8 grams of protein for every pound of body weight. A 130 pound woman would eat 104 grams of protein. This is just an extra scoop or two of whey protein for most women. If your digestive tract can't handle that much, then don't make yourself miserable. Just try to eat as much as protein as you can, remembering that women digest whey and fish easier than steak or chicken.

And when protein becomes the priority, carbs and sugar will take even more of a backseat.

And speaking of sugar and carbs, lets cut a few of those out.

Just like in previous chapters when I discussed the basics of dieting, lets cut something out at the end of the day or late in the day. If you are still eating a cupcake for dessert before you go to bed, stop.

If your last meal of the day usually has pasta or bread or potatoes involved, cut them out.

If you drink a sugary soda in the evening, replace it with a diet soda.

You can keep everything the same, just cut out a few carbs and sugars at the end of the day.

This is step two of Phase I—adjustments to frequency or volume, more protein and fewer carbs and sugars at the end of the day.

Your magic number for reps remains the same. Your time between sets remains the same. We are still tracking, still overloading overtime, still substituting exercises once we plateau.

How long does step two last? Again, as I said at the end of step one, time is a meaningless measure. If the changes in the workout program worked, keep going until you plateau on four exercises. If you were one of the people who had to make some adjustments because your velocity dropped off, I still suggest you stick with step two until you plateau on four exercises.

Most people will go for months on step two and as long as you are getting stronger and building muscle there is no need change the program. Once you plateau, let's move on.

Phase I, Step Three: Dialing In

By now, you may have an absurd lift. Most people are getting close to one at the end of step two of Phase I.

My absurd lift in step two was EZ curls. I had always thought my biceps were a weak or lagging body part. I was wrong. I had just never overloaded them frequently over time with the optimal amount of recovery time. When I started this process of tracking, keeping a log book and overloading over time, I thought 95 pounds was it for me on arm curls. By the end of step two, I was at 120 pounds for 12 reps on the first set. And it just keeps going up.

So, what do we change up in step three?

Diet will be a big change and then we will experiment with volume, frequency and intensity again.

Lets start off with the diet.

After going up in protein and eliminating the night time sugars and carbs, some of you will be seeing the tops of your abs start to peak through.

Protein is and always will be the priority. If you haven't come to believe that at this stage you never will. But hopefully you get it by now.

Remember where you cut out the sugar and carbs in step two? Now, lets move a little bit further counter clockwise if we can. Cut out one more sugary or carby meal or snack or treat.

If you cut out just one more sugary soda, serving of bread, pasta or potatoes, you will see some more muscle start to show up. And, it will probably not affect your strength and muscle gains.

Here is the caveat—those of you who workout in the evening, keep the good carbs late in the day before your workout. If you eat a sandwich, replace the wheat bread with pumpernickel. If you have a potato, try to have a yam. If you drink a sugary soda in the late afternoon, replace it with a diet soda. Just try to cut out the sugar.

Here's the second change. Increase the protein again, this time to 1.5 grams of protein per pound of body weight. If you weigh 170 pounds you would eat 255 grams of protein [170 x 1.5 = 255]. If you weigh 210 pounds you would eat 315 grams of protein [210 x 1.5 = 315].

For women, this is where things get tricky. Women have less testosterone in their blood stream, which means it harder to synthesize protein into muscle, which is why it is harder for women to build muscle than men. Some women can fully utilize up to 1.2 grams of protein per pound of body weight, others top out at .7 grams per pound. Like I said in step two, try eat as much as you can. Spread it out through the day, eating small meals and using whey protein as a snack. Drinking more water and adding a little flax oil helps both men and women handle the increased protein.

Protein is the priority for men and women. And there is a reason we are increasing the protein. We are also going to adjust the workouts.

Back in Part I of the book, there were occasions where the difference between my being stuck on a plateau and making progress was the amount of protein I consumed.

If the overload is increased, but

NITA SPEAKS _____

Women & Protein

Muscle is what makes a beautifully sculpted body. Proteins are the muscle building blocks of your eating plan. Protein should be included at each meal in timing and proportions that make sense for your protein synthesis capabilities, digestive abilities and goals. For women, our protein synthesis capabilities are lower than men because we do not have as much testosterone. Our digestive tracts tend be less capable of processing rough meats like beef, chicken and pork.

I use this equation for women: Eat a half-gram to a full gram per pound of desired lean mass. Take your current body fat percentage, for example we'll use 19 percent and multiply it by your current scale weight of say 135 lbs. [135 x .19 = 25.65]. Subtract the body fat (25.65 lbs.) from your scale weight and you have a lean mass of 109.35 lbs. A woman just wants to maintain would then eat a minimum of 55 grams of protein a day.

If our hypothetical woman from above wants to build up 5 pounds of muscle, she should eat closer to 114 grams of protein a day.

Drink plenty of water, try to get one ounce per pound of scale body weight and plenty of vitamins, especially the sunshine vitamin—vitamin D. If you do not eat enough protein you will lose muscle and not have the long lean sculpted muscles you desire.

there is not enough protein to repair the micro-trauma, you will plateau or even regress. A lot of people go looking for workout solutions, when what they really need is a protein solution.

That said, there are now essentially two general groups of people who have learned a little about their recovery abilities and the workout that can work for them. Some have learned they can make gains with a little more volume or frequency. Others have learned they need more time to recover or make gains with less volume.

Keeping with my desire to control the variables, I suggest taking a few weeks and seeing how the increased protein consumption affects your progress. Then you have some more options to pursue.

As I stated before, the main elements to a workout program are volume, frequency and intensity. A lot of people get hung up on specific exercises, but an exercise is just a way to force the muscle to work and, more importantly, you will eventually plateau on an exercise diminishing its usefulness.

Remember the two general groups from above? Let's start off with the one that needed a little more recovery time. Flip a coin. Heads, you decrease the frequency some more, tails you increase the frequency or volume as suggested back in step two. Some of you who needed a little more recovery time may have actually just needed more protein. The increased protein consumption may allow you to increase the frequency or volume. Or, some of you may be slow healers and adding one more day of recovery time may be what it takes to build muscle.

How can you know for sure? Tracking. Keep track of your lean muscle diameter and your lifts in the gym. Which ever course you decided on, let it run for a few months. If it works, make some slight adjustments to the volume or frequency and see if those adjustments work.

For the group that did well with the increase in frequency or volume, lets increase the volume or frequency again. For those of you who tried Option B, increase the volume by adding one more set to failure. Do the same rotation of Workout #1 and Workout #2, but do three sets instead of just two.

For those who increased the volume by adding an additional set to the old reliable three days a week program, increase the frequency. Instead of taking two days off between Workout #3 and Workout #1, take just one day off.

This may not seem like profound advice, but it is what I missed for years. I could tell you to do Workout X or Workout Z, but how do I know they will work for you? I could tell you to just do some generic workout, but is that what you really need to be doing?

This is what I mean when I say 'Fit for Combat' is a system to find what works for you. By using concrete quantitative measurements like lean muscle diameter and the weights you move in the gym, you can find the volume, frequency and intensity that will allow you to constantly make improvements.

There is no such thing as, 'huge in a hurry'. Everyone is a little different and it takes time to find what works best for you. Sure, you could just try using workouts off the internet or the magazines, and eventually find one that works for you, or you could systematically use quantifiable measurements to find the workout that is nearly perfect for you.

Step three of Phase I should take a long time.

Again, it is based on progress. Some people will like this so much, they stay in it forever, dialing in on the volume, frequency and intensity that works for them and adjusting as their body adapts and that is great.

Seriously, building muscle is fun. Getting stronger is fun. And as Nita said back in step one, a lot of people don't have a body fat problem, they have a lack of muscle problem. A lot of people will achieve their physique goals by just building more muscle, eating more protein and little less sugar.

Here is a rough guide to use to know you are ready to start losing the fat, when you have built a lot of muscle—when you have plateaued on each exercise three times.

For example:

Lets say at the start of step three you were doing flat barbell bench.

You plateau and substitute incline dumbbell bench.

You plateau again and substitute flat dumbbell bench.

You plateau and replace it with incline barbell bench.

Three plateaus. When you have plateaued on every body part three times during step three, you have more than enough muscle to move into Phase II.

Now, some muscle groups will plateau faster than others. You may plateau five or six times on shoulders before you plateau on your legs.

That is just fine.

You want this to last for months and months. You will want to be getting pretty close to heavy duty before you start Phase II. In Phase II you diet. You diet hard. And you will lose muscle. If you don't have a lot of muscle and you diet and lose some muscle, you will look like a scrawny lean guy. You will be weak and stringy and not 'Fit for Combat'. You will definitely not look very good on the beach or at the pool, so what's the point?

If you have to plateau on exercises five times or seven times until you are carrying some real muscle—do it.

Don't be too eager to jump into Phase II until you have built some real muscle.

———————————CHAPTER TWENTY ONE———————————
PHASE II

Phase II, Step One: Lose The Fat

What have we done so far? We've started being systematic in our weight training. Because of our tracking and accountability the muscles have been overloaded over time. After moving through plateaus again and again you have seen that you can move beyond being the average gym goer. Many people after a long stretch in Phase I, are stronger and have more muscle than they ever thought they could.

Your diet has now probably changed as well. You are paying attention to what you eat. You have substituted some sugars and carbs with protein. You have probably come to fully understand that protein is the priority.

If you really stuck with Phase I for months, or even a year, you are a lot bigger and stronger.

Now, lets destroy the last elements of that guy. Get rid of him. Burn him. And burning him is such an apt term.

During what was my personal Phase I, I built myself into a heavy duty machine. But I was tired of being heavy duty. Dragging all that weight around war zones sucked. I was definitely 'Fit (Enough) for Combat' but not truly 'Fit for Combat'.

I needed to get lighter, to lose the fat and keep the muscle.

I tried all kinds of diets and cardio programs and, like the weight lifting programs in the glossy magazines, they didn't work for me. By now we all know the reason why.

The diets in the glossy magazines weren't for guys like us. If Arnold's "Armageddon Arm Workout" doesn't work for us regular guys, why would we think that the "Get Cut Like Conan" diet would work? We have the guts but not the knowledge. We will try anything, but stick with nothing.

Lets take a microscopic look at the eating program portion of this puzzle. If you followed the eating components of Phase I, you have already started it.

See, you have already been sticking with a diet. You didn't even know it. That is the goal of step one of Phase II—to get you following an eating plan.

You have to buy a few devices here so you can properly track your eating and progress:

1. A food scale
2. A set of body fat calipers
3. A cloth measuring tape
4. A bathroom scale (or you can use the one at the gym)

The body fat calipers are not used to measure body fat percentage. Even when done by experienced professionals, the calculation of body fat is fraught with errors. What counts are the millimeters of thickness of fat on your abdominals—specifically on the lower abs where the oblique meets the rectus abdominus and on the upper arm. Remember lean muscle diameter?

A cloth tape to measure your waist, thigh and biceps.

The bathroom scale, though a crude instrument it has its uses.

The most important of the devices is the food scale. You cannot discover the eating plan that works best for you without a food scale.

Back in Phase I, step three, I told you to start eating 1.5 grams of protein per pound of body weight. Question: How many of you really know for sure if you are getting the right amount of protein? Sure, we all know to look at the label and see how many grams of protein there are in a scoop of whey protein. And we can go online and see how many grams of protein there are in an egg, chicken breast, or steak.

But how many of you are measuring the grams of steak and chicken you eat? Be honest.

That is why you need a food scale.

You are not just going to measure how much meat you eat, you are going to measure everything to the gram.

The precision is needed so your eating plan can be tracked and adjusted. You have already seen how effective tracking is in the gym to constantly overload your muscles over time and find the workout plan that works for you. Tracking your diet with that precision will help you underload your diet over time.

The glossy magazines will give a lot of ratios: X% Protein, X% Carbs, X% Sugars, X% Fat. I am sure those are some great general guidelines and they do work, sort of, but they were not designed for you. You need a diet designed specifically for you. All you need to create the diet that burns fat FOR YOU is a food scale and a notebook.

Remember way back in Part I of the book when I started writing down everything I ate and packing my food around in a cooler? Remember the lesson of Lynnie?

You are going to have to start keeping track of everything you eat to the gram and packing your lunches in a cooler.

Yes, it is a lot of work. Yes, it time consuming. But I'm going to give you the same advice Nita Marquez gives her clients, "It is not a question of whether you want to keep track of what you eat, the real question is do you want to be lean or fat?"

Over the course of the next few days, write down everything you eat and drink. Yes, especially everything you drink. Sports

NITA SPEAKS

It is amazing to me the lack of conscience some vendors have when selling food products to people. They are very misleading, but then I guess that would mean that it is our responsibility as the consumers the get educated on the "products" we put into our bodies.

For instance, if I go to a sandwich shop and they say that their bread is whole wheat, which they claim is high in fiber, it could lead me to believe that the sandwich itself is pretty healthy. Well, what they are not telling us that the bread itself, as most bread, contains corn syrup. Then they avoid sharing the reality that the bread is only 2 grams of fiber to 44 grams of carbs, and this pretty much dissolves the value of the fiber.

Given the small amount of protein they are putting on the sandwich (1 oz. of meat maybe), you are pretty much getting a carb and sugar meal, not a protein meal, and it is a carb meal that is so excessive in carbohydrate value, your body cannot metabolize it, so it will turn into sugar, which in excess, turns to fat.

Unless you are running a 10K that day, it is unlikely that your body can avoid the fat storage disaster that the hidden sugars in a sandwich like this can cause to your metabolism and aesthetic balance. Learn about what you eat, you become it. If you are eating too many sugars, even hidden sugars, then it becomes fat. Thus, you become fat.

drinks and juices contain more sugars and carbs than you think. Carbs and sugars are hidden everywhere.

Once you have a few days written down, calculate everything. This will take some time. But remember what Nita said above. If you want to lose the fat, you will do it.

You are calculating total calories, grams of protein, carbs, sugar and fat.

When you get that done, we'll see you in step two of Phase II.

Phase II, Step Two: Counter Clockwise Reduction

You need to know with precision how many calories grams of protein, carbohydrates, sugars and fats you eat on average day.

If you do not know, go back and do step one of Phase II again.

If you do not know exactly what you are eating, it is difficult to determine what you need to change in your diet to lose fat. You will not be able to under load your food intake over time.

This step is about working through a system to help you find your diet. That's right, your customized diet, just for you. It's a diet you can tweak and manipulate as your physique and goals evolve. Instead of just telling you what to eat, I am going to show you a system you can use to become your own personal eating plan guru.

We all hear people say, "It is just so hard to eat right."

Bull. It is easier to eat right than eat crap if you follow a simple plan. Let me illustrate.

How many of you are self-sustaining farmers or gardeners?

If you are not either of these, then you buy your food. You have to make a conscious decision what to buy. Eating properly to lose fat and build muscle is not about eating, it is about buying. If you don't buy crappy food, you can't eat crappy food.

It is easy to eat right if you don't buy a bunch of junk. So, when you are at the grocery store, don't buy it. If you are at a restaurant, don't order it.

That is really all there is to it. It gets even easier when you start eating basically the same things every day. In the early steps here, it will be easier for you if you eat the same foods five or six days a week. That will eliminate a lot of questions and a lot of variables. What you want to do is establish a baseline of some sort. Yes, your body will adapt to that baseline of what you eat, which is just fine. If you are still gradually building muscle, the caloric expenditure will always be gradually going up. But why we really want to establish a baseline is so that we can start underloading what you eat.

And this is the crucible decision. A lot you are going to complain, "but I like variety, I don't want to eat the same boring foods every day like oats, yams, vegetables, eggs, fish, steak. I want flavor and texture. Yada, yada, yada."

When you say that, what you are actually saying is that you still want to be fat. Remember what Lynnie said? "I would love to be able to eat cheesecake and chocolate and still look this way, but I can't. Tight glutes and abs or cheesecake? No brainer for me."

If you want the crap food more than you want abs, there is nothing neither myself nor Nita can do for you.

Nita is gonna try and motivate you a bit, but

NITA SPEAKS _____

You want muscle, you want energy, and you want your best overall symmetry. Getting to the gym is half the battle. When you are taking on the challenges of your workouts with fortitude and vigor, eating the right things doesn't seem so hard. There is something more plausible in eating healthy once you have just ripped your muscles to shreds breaking your body down through an insane workout in the free weights section of your gym.

We all feel more powerful once we have thrown the weights around to show that we own it! We are unconquerable and pretty much feel like we can do whatever the hell we want once we break down our bodies this way.

Then there is the other guy, who sat on his ass watching TV, and eating Cheese Puffs and pie. Which one do you want to be?

after that it is all up to you. It is ultimately your decision.

If you are still thinking that you want cupcakes or pizza or sub sandwiches more than you want abs—implement what you are willing to. Even following a few of the principles will make difference.

If you have decided that abs are more important than a bunch of junk, lets get you on an eating plan.

Write it out so it looks something like my current eating plan below:

Protein 315 grams
Carbs 64 grams
Sugar 10 grams

3:00 a.m. (midnight snack if I wake up hungry)
Whey protein shake with water
18 Grams protein
2 grams sugar

6:00 a.m.
Whey Protein shake with water, 1 Amino Acid Tab, 2 Glutamine Caps
18 Grams Protein
2 Grams Sugar

6:30 a.m.
Sprints

7:00 a.m.
1 Cup Oatmeal (80 grams) with two scoops whey powder and Flax Oil
20 Grams Protein
52 Grams Carbohydrate
4 Grams Sugar

9:30 a.m.
8 Egg whites, 3 yolk
33g Protein
2g carbs

12:00 p.m.
Steak meal with broccoli
170 grams steak
315 Cal
45g protein
3g carbs
1 Amino Acid Tab, 2 Glutamine Caps

1:00 p.m.
Lift Weights

2:30 p.m.
Whey Protein Shake 2 scoops
36 Grams Protein
4 Grams Sugar

4:30 p.m.
8 Egg whites, 3 yolk
155 Cal
33g Protein
2g carbs

7:00 p.m.
8 Egg whites, 3 yolk
155 Cal
33g Protein
2g carbs

9:00 p.m.
170 grams steak
45g protein
1 Amino Acid Tab, 2 Glutamine Caps

10:00 p.m.
Go to Bed

On Wednesday, I eat a huge green salad

Saturday, I do a crazy cheat eating all kinds of crap

I literally eat the same way five days a week. On Wednesday I'll throw in the huge green salad with a balsamic vinegar and oil dressing. On Saturday, I go crazy. I still get all my protein in because protein is always the priority. But I will have pizza, tacos, cupcakes. Whatever strikes my fancy.

But I didn't always eat this way. Back when I was heavy duty, I ate like this.

6:00 a.m.
Wake up
Whey Protein Drink
150 Cal
27 g Protein
2 g carbs
Glutamine caps

6:30 a.m.
Cardio

7:30 a.m.
Meal Replacement Drink--
350 Cal
32 g Protein
12 g Carbs
With Flax oil

9:45 a.m.
5 Jumbo eggs with cheese
5 whites, 1 Yolk
155 Cal
27 g Protein
2 g carbs
14 g cheese
3.5 g protein
1 g carb

11:00 a.m.
Chicken meal
150 g charcoal grilled chicken breast
75 g sweet potato
35 g broccoli
14 g cheese
390 Calories
45 g protein
16.75 g carbs

12:00 p.m.
Meal Replacement Drink
350 cal
32 g protein
12 g carbs

1:00 p.m.
Lift weights

2:30 p.m.
Meal Replacement Drink
350 Cal
32 g Protein
12 g carbs
Glutamine caps

4:00 p.m.
Chicken meal
150 g charcoal grilled chicken breast
75 g sweet potato
35 g broccoli
14 g cheese
390 Calories
45 g protein
16.75 g carbs

6:30 p.m.
chicken meal
150 g charcoal grilled chicken breast
75 g sweet potato
35 g broccoli
14 g cheese

9:00 p.m.
another chicken meal

10:00 p.m.
Go to bed

3:00 a.m.
Midnight snack
Whey protein
150 Cal
27 g Protein
2 g carbs

Total Per Day
Protein 357 g
Carbs 120 g

Notice the difference? These days I take in way less carbs and sugars and no pre-processed meal replacement drinks.

My eating plan back when I was heavy duty was not a bad plan. In fact, it is a really good plan for building a lot of muscle and strength. But, it was a horrible plan for my goal of losing fat. The only upside to it was the consistency. I had everything written out and followed it consistently. That allowed me to make very precise adjustments and track the results over the course of weeks and months. You need to have everything listed and measured on your base eating plan so you can make the same adjustments.

One of the biggest mistakes people make when trying to lose fat is going 'all-in' on the diet from day one. They have no idea what they are eating, they have no idea what their base diet is. They find some diet on-line or in a magazine or a book and decide to do it.

When you drastically cut calories, sugars and carbs you will lose some weight, maybe even quite a bit of fat, but after a few weeks your body will adapt. If you went 'all-in' from day one, there is nothing else eliminate and the fat loss will come to a halt.

Our goal here is to maximize the fat loss from each underload in calories, carbs and sugars by gradually eliminating them. I call this underload over time.

Once you know, with precision, what you are eating, you can start tweaking, experimenting, modifying, substituting and tracking the results.

Take a look at your list of meals and snacks. What is the easiest thing to eliminate or substitute? For me, the first thing I cut out was the sweet potato from the 9:00 p.m. meal. I did not need those carbs for right before I went to sleep. After two weeks, I didn't see much change. Instead of getting discouraged I cut the sweet potato out of the 6:30 p.m. meal. After two weeks, I started to notice something. I was a few pounds lighter. And the top of my abs became a little more visible.

Now I'm motivated. So, I cut out the sweet potato at the 4:00 p.m. meal. I get two pounds lighter and my waist was a bit smaller.
You see the pattern? See how I was working backward through my day? See how I did it slowly over the course of weeks?

This is the key to discovering your own personal eating plan. The plan that works for you.

Start at the end of the day and gradually eliminate sugars and carbs. This is the under load over time. In this step, you will keep underloading until you reach your fat loss goal.

The other thing that can happen is you underload to a point where it is no longer compatible with your lifestyle, but are still not at your fat loss goal (how we deal with that is a series of ways to play tricks on your body which are explained in subsequent chapters). For now, the short answer is if you get to a point where the lack of carbs affects your ability to concentrate, work and be a productive member of society, add in a few more carbs and call that your new base diet.

A lot of people fail at dieting because they try to go cold turkey. This is a mistake for two reasons. When you go cold turkey your body will rebel. You will get carb/sugar deprivation headaches. You will feel sluggish. You will give up.

The second problem with going cold turkey is the Krebs cycle, the body's metabolism will adjust to the rapid under load. Once that adjustment is complete, fat loss will stop.

Gradual under load is the key. This is not a diet, this about discovering an eating plan that allows you to burn fat and maintain as much muscle as possible.

Tracking is the key

With your food scale, you know how much you are eating and can adjust the carbs back slowly.

The body fat calipers are used to measure the thickness of fat. The tape measure is to track the size of your thigh, waist and biceps. The scale, your overall weight. Your training log will show you whether you are getting stronger (building muscle), staying the same or losing muscle (getting weaker). Using the millimeters of fat thickness on your upper arm and the circumference of your upper arm, you continue to track lean tissue diameter.

You want to track the trends. Are the millimeters of fat thickness going down? Is your lean tissue staying the same? Are you weighing less? Is your waist/thigh/ bicep smaller? How is your strength?

As a general rule, the most important measurement is the thickness of fat where the oblique merges with the rectus abdominals (just a few inches to the left or right of you navel) and lean tissue diameter. If the millimeters of thickness are getting smaller, you are losing fat. If they are staying the same over the course of weeks, but everything else is trending down, you are losing muscle.

If you are underloading and losing muscle but not fat, the ketosis outlined in the next chapter may be what you need. Or, it is time to do a metabolic reset as will be discussed in Chapter 22.

For most people the gradual underload will work great. As you work counter-clockwise through the day eliminating sugars and carbs over the course of weeks and months, you will lose a few pounds of fat a month.

If you follow it all the way through to its logical end, you could find yourself just eating a bowl of oatmeal or some other low-sugar carbs for breakfast as your total carbohydrate intake. You may also find a new baseline eating plan for yourself.

My current eating plan listed previously in this chapter is my base eating plan. What I mean by that is, it's an eating plan that allows me to build muscle, strength and stamina and train to be "Fit for Combat" without gaining fat. As I gradually build more muscle, I can eat a few more grams of oatmeal for breakfast without gaining fat. On the other side of the equation, I can lose fat by eating a few less grams of oatmeal.

It is my hope that most of the people reading this book will be able to achieve their fat loss goals through the gradual underload. If you get where you want to be, through the underload, stick with that eating plan or maybe add in a few more carbs. It is likely to be your base eating plan.

But what if you want more? If you want more, if you want to get really lean, then take the plunge into step three.

Phase II, Step Three: The Final Pounds

I looked like crap. Seriously. And I felt like crap. All you could say about me was that I was getting really lean. My muscles were small and flat. My strength was plummeting.

Welcome to ketosis. I don't want to scare you off, I just want you to know what you are getting into—especially for a first timer. It will not be fun, you really won't even like what you see in the mirror. But after you are done and get back to your base diet—whomp!

If you thought you hit an identity crises before in this system, you ain't seen nothing yet. Which is why it is important to keep your eyes on the prize. The ketogenic carb cycling is not an end in itself. It is temporary. It is just a technique to get where you want to be.

When you get to the end of the ketogenic carb cycling road and get back to your base diet, people will start asking you if you compete in bodybuilding contests. People will think you are a bodybuilder. The women who followed this system will start to look like a fitness model or figure competitor after the ketosis. Some people will not even recognize you.

Now, not everyone has to do this. If you have six pack after Phase I or after Step One and Two of Phase II, I hate you. Really, I do. But hate does not get us a six pack. Ketosis does. More accurately, the decision to go all in for about two months or as long as you can put up with it.

Lets start off easy like I did back in Chapter 15 and how I explained underload in step two of Phase II. If you remember, I still had carbs in my eating plan at around 11:00 a.m. I got rid of those carbs. I also substituted all the chicken with steak or eggs.

Protein is the priority right. And in this step since all we eat is protein you have to get it from the best sources that your body can use.

Just by improving the quality of your protein and getting down to one carb meal you should have gotten quite a bit leaner and your muscles may have gotten a tad-bit harder. If that gets you to where you want to be. Viola. Welcome to your base diet. You may need to add back a little extra carbs BUT NOT SUGAR before your workout, but you have probably got it.

The rest of us, let's keep going.

So, what carbs do you have left to manipulate? If you have worked your way counter clockwise through the day eliminating all the carbs and sugars, the only thing left after a few months will be breakfast. If you are still eating something like a corn based breakfast cereal, switch to one cup (80 grams) of oatmeal for breakfast.

If you are going all out on the Saturday cheat—pizza, sugary soda, cupcakes, etc., cut it back by 50 percent for two weeks. Keep track of what you eat on the Saturday cheat. After two weeks, you will have lost some more fat. Okay, cut it by 50 percent again. Not a whole lot of cheating left now.

The goal is to get your cheat meal to just an extra bowl of oatmeal and a large green salad.

At this point, there are only three types of people. Those who through this intense underload have achieved their goals, those want to get almost contest ripped and people like me who have to fight hard to lose fat.

NITA SPEAKS

When you are on a ketogenic diet, two things are obvious. First, you will be low on energy because of the lack of carbohydrates. Secondly, you will have a harder time breaking down your food because of the lack of fiber in your diet that results from lack of carbs.

Some key points to choosing your protein staples for each meal: The protein in red meat is so hard to break down, you don't want this to be your only source. Although the red meat is high in iron and definitely gives you an energy boost, it is not readily available protein, especially without the intestinal aid of certain carbs to break it down and assimilate it during digestion. Therefore, you will want to limit yourself to five servings per week if you are doing a no-carb diet. Furthermore, you will want to take in poultry because of the fat concentration for its energy source as well. The best food, while you will still want to regulate possible mercury ingestion, is fish, which is rich in Omega-three fats and much easier to break down as a food to assimilate protein into your muscles. Salmon and sea bass tend to carry much higher fat contents than white fish, but white fish tend to be easier to break down and assimilate in digestion.

Egg whites are very easily assimilated and contain some sodium. Whey, egg whites and soy protein when in liquid or powder form are readily assimilated, but again, do not enhance energy as well as higher fat proteins. Also, when doing these diets, it's important to remember that you need incredible amounts of water (1 ounce per pound of body weight at least) and Vitamin D for the protein synthesis to avoid protein buildup.

There is only one thing left to manipulate—morning oatmeal. And now we are heading into ketosis.

If you are a total masochist cut it all out at once. If you are not into masochism, drop your 80 grams of oats by 20 grams each week.

If, after three weeks you are still not where you want to be—welcome to three or four days of insanity followed by a longer stretch of a different kind of mania. Step four is a wild ride.

Phase II, Step Four: Crazy Ketosis

What we are going to do here is one half rocket science one half 30-year-old science.

Everyone has probably heard of Dr. Atkins. We are going to use a variant of the old tried and true Atkins diet. Actually, if you have followed the plan, you have been on it for some time.

Okay, the Saturday cheat is down to an extra bowl of oatmeal and a salad. We are down to 20 grams of oatmeal in the morning.

You need to buy one more tool. Go to the pharmacy and buy some keto test strips. They are behind the counter but anyone can buy them. Read the instructions on the box of the keto strips. Pretty straight forward.

The keto strips are important because they will tell you whether or not you are in Ketosis. What is Ketosis? When your body is burning Ketones as fuel. What are Ketones?

Glad you asked. Ketones are fat that have been 'cracked' into betahydroxybutyric acids and acetoacetic acids.

It's a little confusing but, here is what you really need to know. Ketones are used by the body as fuel when the glycogen (sugar/carbs) is taken away and maintenance calories remain the same.

If the body has no glycogen to fuel the brain and other functions, it releases glucogen. Glucogen in the liver converts fat to Ketones which the body and brain will use for energy.

When you are ketogenic your body is burning fat for fuel. Not just some fat, not just a little fat, it is primarily burning fat for fuel. Pretty cool. Obviously this is the best way to get the remaining fat off. It is also a great diet for just about anyone—which is why Dr. Atkins was a mega millionaire.

But there is one major drawback. The first three to five days absolutely suck. Most people fail on the Atkins diet or any type of a ketogenic diet within 48 hours. Why? Because before the body starts releasing glucogen to turn fat into Ketones you will feel like crap. You will have the worst headache. You will have no energy. You will not be able to think. You will be a zombie.

Nita is one of the toughest people I know, and even after all these years of training and eating properly and doing ketogenic diets for fitness contests, the first few days still throw her for a loop.

The more carbs and sugars your body is used to getting, the worse the initial shock is. Which is why I like to ease into it a little bit.

But, once your body starts producing ketones, you will feel much better. People have different reactions to ketosis. Some people never feel 100 percent. Some people get manic and experience insomnia. Some experience a mild euphoria. And some people feel like crap the whole time.

I get a little manic and euphoric and my brain power drops a little bit. If you have a supra-genius IQ, you will not notice the loss in brain power. The rest of us mortals will notice it. Making lists, taking notes and calendar reminders become essential during ketosis.

If you can make it past the first three to five days, the rest of the cycle is easy. The second time you do it, it is even easier. I recently did a ketogenic cycle and only had a headache for one day, then the mania kicked in. On the fifth day I felt "wobbly". My brain worked but I just felt odd. On the sixth day, I felt absolutely normal.

Now we've all seen low carb diet failures. Why do they fail? For the same reason that guy never makes any progress in the gym.

Like I said, most people don't make it past 48 hours. Those who stay on Atkins or South Beach for a long stretch lose fat. But what happens when they stop? They go back to their crappy, sugary, carby eating habits that made them fat in the first place.

And at some point the body does figure out what is going on, adapts and the dieters plateau.

The path to ketosis is easy if you have your eating plan worked out. All you are doing is substituting your remaining carbs with protein and your whey protein with a whey that has zero sugars. Most whey protein powders have 2 grams of sugars per serving, find one that has zero grams of sugar. Eggs and meat have just trace sugars. If you sneak in even a few grams of sugar this whole process fails and all you will have to show for it is a headache.

You want to stay steady on the calories.

For your weight lifting, stick with the basic program. If you feel run down, cut your sets back from three to two but still lift as hard as you can. I would not recommend much cardio during this. If you are doing cardio, cut it in half. Train like you normally would, maintain the pattern, keep your log book.

Ready to go? Good. Lets work this one through by the numbers. I use a 12 day ketogenic carb cycle. Some experts recommend ten, others seven. I like 12. If I'm gonna be ketogenic, I say let the good times roll. Here's an example of what works for me:

Day 1 Saturday
Your cheat meal should be down to some extra oatmeal and a salad and do what you normally do on Saturday.

Day 2 Sunday
No carbs, no sugars. Replace any remaining carbs with a protein source of equal calories. You will feel like crap today.

Day 3 Monday
Same as Sunday.

Day 4 Tuesday
Same as Monday

Day 5 Wednesday
Eat the same as Tuesday. Use your keto strips a few times during the day. Did they turn color? Are you Ketogenic? Some people will be ketogenic by now. Some will not.

Day 6 Thursday
Eat the same as Wednesday. Use your keto strips. Most everyone will be getting some ketones in their system by now. Many of you will start to feel better.

Day 7 Friday
Same as Thursday.

Day 8 Saturday
Same as Friday, but if you want to have a ketogenic cheat day, give it a shot. How do you have ketogenic cheat day? By eating a lot of fat. Pork rinds, bacon, sausage. Be careful on the sausage as many types contain sugars. The ketogenic cheat day breaks the monotony of the eating plan and keeps the body from adapting to the relatively constant caloric intake.

Day 9 Sunday
Back on the usual ketogenic diet. If you did the cheat, your keto strips test will show a higher concentration of ketones.

Day 10 Monday
Same as Sunday

Day 11 Tuesday
Same as Monday

Day 12 Wednesday
You can have carbs again in the manner listed below for the next 48 hours

You will be eating every two hours for the next 48 hours. The closer you can get to eating every two hours the better. Really, get up in the middle of the night and eat. Here is what your carb re-feed plan should look like:

Meals 1-4: Fruit juice with whey protein, a big glass of it.
Meals 5-9: 50% Fruit juice, 50% water with whey protein in the big glass. Some type of breakfast cereal made from corn.
Meals 10-14: Steak, sweet potatoes, vegetables, oatmeal and a shot of fruit juice.
Meals 15-18: Steak, sweet potatoes, vegetables, oatmeal, pasta, no fruit juice.
Meals 19-24: 25% fruit juice, 75% water with whey protein in the big glass.

Then you repeat the cycle starting at the second day with no carbs.

Some people will show barely a trace of ketones on the test strips. That is fine. Remember, the test strips show ketones in the urine stream, exiting the body. These are the ketones that have not been used for energy. If you are lifting hard and active, most of the ketones will be used for energy. If you want to test if you are ketogenic, eat some pork rinds or a lot of fat and wait a few hours to use your test strips again. The color change should be noticeable.

How many times do you go through this cycle? One or two times is enough for most people. I did three of them.

At the end of the two days of carbs, you should 'whomp' in size. Your muscles will be full, round and looking 300 percent better than you did on Day number 11.

That will be motivation enough to give it another run or two. And you might get into ketosis a bit quicker. Since you know what to expect from the carb crash, it won't be nearly as painful.

If you are done with ketogenic carb cycling do not make the mistake and start eating like an idiot. Go through the 48 hour carbohydrate marathon then get back on a base diet with slightly less carbs than your normal base diet. If I am not going to do another run of ketosis, I do not do the super carbohydrate refeed—my body's insulin reaction to sugar would want to turn it all into fat—so I just get back on the base diet.

This is where you really, really need to put the fat calipers to work. If you see any (and I mean any) unwanted upward trend cut back on the carbs. It might be as simple as reducing your morning carbs by 10 or 20 grams.

If you are using the scale, using the fat calipers, tracking your lean tissue diameter and measuring all your food you can maintain a relatively low body fat permanently.

As I said before, this is all about you calculating the perfect diet for you.

Go back to having a quality cheat on Saturday. A few people can even get away with a Saturday afternoon/evening/night through Sunday at noon cheat. If you are not that person, you know what do to. Gradually cut back.

It will take some time to find your personalized eating plan. The key is that you now know how to do it by following the steps and principles outlined above and consistently tracking what you eat and results OVER TIME. *This is not a diet, this is an eating plan you can use for the rest of your life.*

CHAPTER TWENTY TWO
PHASE III MAINTENANCE AND SLOW REBUILDING

I bumped into that guy at the gym.

I was doing dumbbell rows. A great big heavy duty guy, John, was on the bench next to me. That guy came up to John and asked him something about traps.

John, like I said, is heavy duty. Big guns, huge chest, tall traps and good sized belly. But he's in his 40s and is retired from the Army. Heavy duty works for him and he follows the basics of overload over time.

John was showing him the finer points of shrugs—a concept totally lost on me— when that guy asks me about my three ring binder and why I write a number in it after every set.

I finished the exercise out, took a sip of water and gave him the 30 second explanation. He was skeptical. A few days later, he asked me again. I saw him yesterday and he was keeping a log book. Nice.

Phase III is the final burial of the old mentalities. Until now things have moved rapidly. Yeah, yeah, I know, it may have taken you a year or more to get here, but that is light speed compared to this, because Phase III is forever.

In Phase I you built a lot of strength and muscle. That was pretty fun. Phase II was tougher with the controlled eating plans but the results were fun. But you are not as big or strong as you were at the end of Phase I. That kinda sucks.

At the end of Phase II, I told you to get back on your maintenance diet, track everything and pay close attention to the calipers.

The goal of Phase III, and I think the goal of the rest of your life, is to stay as lean as you can while still making muscle and strength gains.

In Phase I the strength and muscle may have came fast. Here in Phase III it will come slowly, but because you are lean, every gain in muscle will be more visible.

It is almost impossible for a person to gain muscle and lose fat in Phase III. It is not impossible, but exceedingly difficult to gain muscle without gaining fat, or, more precisely, without gaining much fat.

When a person first starts training they can build muscle and lose fat. You can build muscle and lose fat in Phase I. You will be able to gain some strength and muscle quickly at the start of Phase III, but it will start to slow down.

So, do we change things, do we go looking for the silver bullet solution in a glossy magazine? Actually, at this phase, you might get some innovative ideas from a glossy magazine. But the principles still apply. Overload over time, tracking, accountability, controlled eating plan.

When coming out of the Phase II ketogenic carb cycling, or one of the less drastic steps you must be meticulous with your eating plan. Weigh everything. Stick with the plan. Protein is the priority. Add carbs back slowly in the morning. Don't eat sugar. I tell people all the time I'm allergic to sugar. I love sugar, but I am allergic to it—it makes me fat.

If you are using your calipers, and you see the millimeters of thickness start to trend upward then cut back the carbs a little, just a little. Or, tame down the Saturday cheat.

At this stage you are your own diet expert. If you want to experiment, experiment. But, just experiment the way a scientist would—with meticulously tracking.

Personally, I'm not much into experimenting that much with the diet. I found what works for me and I'm sticking to it.

The weight training and cardio—I will experiment with those in very precise and controlled manner by tracking my lean tissue diameter and gains in my log book.

This is where you really start finding the workout program that works for you and apply the core principles of the 'Fit for Combat' system.

——————— CHAPTER TWENTY THREE ———————
THERE IS NO SUCH THING AS AVERAGE

This chapter is the thesis of the 'Fit for Combat' system. It is the most important chapter as it lays out the guiding principles behind everything I have suggested. It is also the road map to help you understand why I would rather show you a system of quantifiable measurements and how to think about them, rather than just tell you to do something.

I put it this late in the book because it would probably blow your mind if it was the first chapter and you didn't get to see how I applied the principles and measurements and how to apply them in your own effort to build muscle and lose fat.

The human body is incredibly durable. It repairs itself, it adapts and even learns. It also responds to certain biological laws.

When those laws are tested and measured in an experiment or controlled study there is an average. That average becomes the rule, the standard. More often than not, the standard becomes the standard because it fits rather nicely into normal distribution—the bell curve.

Look at the chart below:

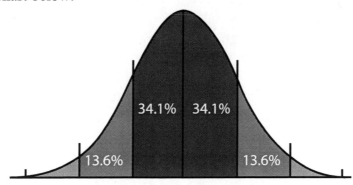

This is the standard bell curve. It is absolutely stunning sometimes how much of human activity, behavior and physiology falls within the standard bell curve. There will always be an "average" but the mathematical concept of normal distribution plots the ranges where people fall in the average. Just about every time, people will be within one standard deviation from the average—the 34.1% to the left or right of the average. Or, to say it another way, 68.2 percent of the population will be pretty close to average.

If we were to apply this to muscular hypertrophy, 68.2 percent of the men in America would be fairly close in their hypertrophy abilities. There will be smaller numbers on the right with more capability for hypertrophy and smaller numbers on the left with less capability for hypertrophy.

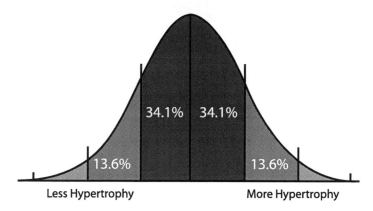

The basic old reliable three exercises, three times a week weight lifting plan I suggested you start with in step one of Phase I hits somewhere in the 68.2 percent.

The people on the far right side of the curve will benefit from any—and I mean any—overload weight lifting program. The people on the left benefit best from programs that inflict less micro-trauma with less frequency.

This is the genius of the low rep, low volume high-intensity programs. They are going to work for everyone, especially beginners, which is why so many people, including me, advocate it. The great error is in assuming that since high intensity generally works for everyone, everyone should do it.

But because it is almost guaranteed to work, I suggest people start with it then add volume and frequency until they find with precision what works for them.

The human body is durable, it adapts, it learns, but it is also a precision machine. Each human body is a custom, precision machine and each workout plan should be adapted and customized for each individual person.

Each person has their own hypertrophy zone—the optimal overload/micro-trauma/recovery zone.

The true goal of the 'Fit for Combat' system is to find your hypertrophy zone, the amount of overload your body can recover from over time—time and time again. The goal is to find the workout program with the amount of intensity, volume and frequency that, when combined with a sustainable eating plan, allows you to gradually build muscle while maintaining a relatively low body fat.

We've long since given up guessing at anything. Workouts are logged and tracked. Food is weighed and measured. Finding your hypertrophy zone requires the same kind of measuring and tracking.

The tools are our trusty notebook, a cloth tape measure, a pair of body fat calipers and a healthy dose of time and patience.

The weight lifting log book will tell you if you are getting stronger, but is the strength gain from muscle or myelin tissue?

Myelin tissue is the fatty sheath that surrounds nerves. The more myelin, the more efficient the nerves are at firing. The more efficient the nerves, the faster and more powerful the muscle contractions. The nerves become more adept at firing in sequence. This is why golfers and tennis players practice their swing. Repetition builds the myelin tissue. This is also known as muscle memory.

If the nerves play such a large role in athletic moves, and since a bench press is very athletic move involving multiple muscles and balance, how much of an increase one's performance on the bench press is due to muscle or myelin?

Some people would guess. I prefer to measure and measure over the course of time. This measurement is how you find your hypertrophy zone. This measurement is the lean tissue diameter I first mentioned back in Chapter 3 and constantly referenced in previous chapters.

The cloth tape measure will tell you the circumference of the upper arm. A crude measurement at best, but one that works.

The fat calipers measure the millimeters of thickness of subcutaneous fat.

Other than an increase in the size of the humerus, the bone of the upper arm, the size of the arm is determined by the thickness of fat, the size of the bicep and the size of the tricep.

Over the course of time, if the millimeters of fat thickness as measured by the calipers remains the same and the circumference increases, you are building muscle.

If the millimeters and circumference remain the same, but your lifts continue to improve, the myelin is the source of the strength gain (not a bad thing if you are power lifter).

The difficult part is if the millimeters of fat thickness are increasing and the circumference is increasing. Now, some people would just be happy guessing that because their arms were getting bigger they were building muscle. But as you have noticed, this system is not about guessing. And with a little math, we won't have to guess.

Ready for a rough application of high school geometry? And I do mean rough. There are more accurate measurements, but this will get us pretty close. Yep, we are going to use the mathematical constant of pi or 3.14.

Lets assume for a minute that your upper arm is perfect circle rather than an odd oval.

This perfect circle of an upper arm is 430 millimeters (43 centimeters) in circumference, which means the diameter of the arm is 136.9 mm.

430/pi = diameter, 136.9 mm

If the thickness of subcutaneous fat is 6 mm, the diameter of the lean tissue is 130.9. With this number you have a quantifiable way to track muscle gains. And if you are not quantifying you are guessing and if you are guessing you might as well be rolling dice.

Lets track this over time.

January 1st
Overall Circumference: 430 mm
Fat thickness from skin fold calipers: 6 mm

430 mm / 3.14 = 136.9 mm

136.9 mm – 6 mm = 130.9

The actual formula would be:

(C/pi) – t= L

On February 1st
Overall Circumference: 445 mm
Fat thickness from skin fold calipers: 8 mm

(445/3.14) – 8=

445 mm/3.14 = 141.7 mm

141.7mm – 8mm = 133.7

Or an increase in the lean tissue diameter of 2.8 mm! That 2.8mm increase is a .021 increase or, an increase of 2.1%. These percentage changes are important to track over time as well.

As long as the lean tissue diameter is increasing, you are doing something right and somewhere in the range of your hypertrophy zone.

If your lean tissue diameter is staying the same, you are not in your hypertrophy zone. If your lean tissue diameter is decreasing, you may be doing something drastically wrong.

To dial in on your hypertrophy zone takes measurements like this over the course of months, even years. If you are satisfied with the range of the zone you are in, keep on keeping on. If you are not in your zone, or want to dial in even closer to achieve optimal results, it is time to experiment.

Lets go back to the bell curve.

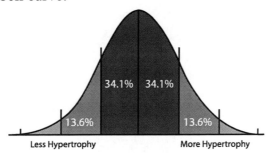

The people on the far left probably know who they are. The people on the far right probably know who they are. After Phase I, you have a really good idea of where you are.

The guys on the far right are already muscular. The guys on the far left tend to be scrawny and lanky. Those on the far right should add more volume, more failure sets and frequency to increase the overload. The guys on the far left should decrease volume, decrease frequency and do fewer failure sets and decrease the overload.

But, for the 68.2 percent in the middle, just flip a coin. Heads you slightly increase the overload, tails you slightly decrease the overload. This slight increase could be just one more or one less failure set per workout or exercise, or an increase or decrease of frequency of just a day.

If this sounds familiar, it is exactly what I advised in Phase I.

Continue to track the changes in lean tissue circumference for a few months.

If the lean tissue diameter stays the same, you know the change was incorrect. If it decreases, you know the change was really incorrect. If it increases, it may be what you need.

For the people who get an increase over the course of months, there comes an important question? Did the rate of the increase, the regular percentage change, go up or down?

If it went up, you may be moving to your optimal zone. If it went down, you may need to back off a bit. Also, be aware that gains do diminish over time. The first gains come the easiest and fastest.

For example, lets look at our 2.1% gain from above.

From January to February our test subject increased the lean tissue circumference by 2.1%. Similar gains in lean tissue diameter over time would yield the following:

March: 136.5mm	2.8mm gain
April: 139.4mm	2.8mm gain
May: 142.3mm	2.9mm gain
June: 145.3mm	2.9mm gain
July: 148.3mm	3.0mm gain

You see the problem here. Even if you gain 2.1% in lean tissue circumference every month, for a few months, you would go from 16.8 inches to 18.14 inches.

Sorry kids, it ain't gonna happen. Does not work like that forever.

What is more likely to happen over the course of time is, for the percentage gains to gradually decrease. There will still be increases in the lean tissue circumference, but the changes will be small and not occur month to month but over the course of months. What you want to look for in your experimentation is a huge drop off in percentage change that coincides with a change in frequency or volume.

Over time, the gains in lean muscle are measured in millimeters a year. If that discourages you, try this visualization: flex your bicep and stack five dimes on top of it. Now imagine those five dimes added to your quads, chest, delts, etc. Even millimeters can make a large visual impact.

When you get into your hypertrophy zone, you will be making gradual increases over the course of months. If you are not making gradual increases in lean tissue circumference, you are not in your zone and either over training or way under training.

Over training is easy to understand—the overload and micro-trauma on the muscle is more than can be recovered from before the next workout. It is also exacerbated by poor nutrition and not eating enough protein.

Under training can happen as well. Under training is when the muscle is not being overloaded enough to induce hypertrophy or, the frequency between workouts is too long and the catabolic window opens and is often exacerbated by poor nutrition.

The human body will gladly use protein for fuel. Some bodies seem to prefer their own skeletal muscle to any other fuel.

If you are under training, your body is not getting the signals to repair the micro-trauma and will gladly go on its normal catabolic path and achieve a steady state, no muscle growth or a gradual reduction of muscle. The myelin tissue increase will often mask any loss of muscle or zero muscle gain.

This is why you need to experiment with the overload over time and track the lean tissue circumference.

Does this sound like a lot work? It shouldn't. The whole process of measuring, writing, doing the math and tracking only takes a few minutes a month.

Through gradual experimentation you can find the workout system that is perfectly tailored for you. Now, you could try to guess. You could cobble together a workout from the glossy magazines or the internet. But those workouts are not specifically designed for you.

The only way to find the perfect workout for you is to experiment and track the results. The difference between being in your optimal hypertrophy zone and over training could be a few sets.

Once you are in your zone, you will make constant progress. It will be gradual progress, but it is better than guessing and never making any progress.

Over the years I've used this system to find a workout a workout that works for me. But some people would call my personal workout heresy. On the internet, in books and magazines there are fierce advocates for all kinds of training systems.

Here is the absolute truth, and it is revealed by the bell curve.

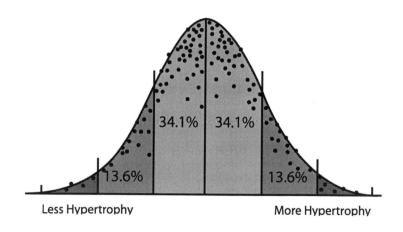

Less Hypertrophy   More Hypertrophy

Every single workout program no matter how hare brained is going to work really well for some percentage of the population. Notice how there are a lot of dots in this one. Each dot represents where one person falls on the hypertrophy scale. Even though there are 68 dots clumped up near the average, none of them are in exactly the same position. Even a little difference between hypertrophy abilities can yield remarkably different results—especially over the course of months and years.

The same thing applies to the eating plan.

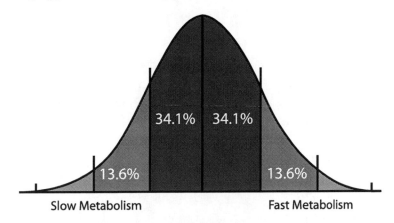

34.1%   34.1%

13.6%   13.6%

Slow Metabolism   Fast Metabolism

Here again, 68 percent of the population will be fairly close. There will be the average or the standard, but they are not the same. Even a difference in metabolic rate of 50 calories a day begins to add up over the course of a few months.

Just like the training plan, the eating plan has to be specifically for you.

I could grab 100 guys at the gym at random, put them on an insane high frequency, high volume program and for two of them it would be their perfect workout. For another 13 of them, it would be a pretty good plan. Another 35 would have marginal gains at best. But for the remaining 50, it wouldn't work at all.

This is why most training and diet plans on the internet or in a book or magazine are a crock. If you ever come across someone who swears there is only one perfect workout or diet, look them in the eye and say, "Yes, there is only one perfect workout for each individual person and it changes as they change."

As you build more muscle, grow older, become more fit, the workout that works best for you will change. The same with your metabolism and eating plan.

But the principles never change. The Rosenfield principle is universal. Overload over time works every time. The intensity, volume and frequency of the overload and your eating plan is what has to be adapted.

My workout program has evolved over the years. Some people think it is the stupidest workout they have ever seen. Some people can't believe I can do so little yet still improve. But, it is what is working for me right now. The proof is in how I perform in combat zones, what I see in the mirror and the back flap of this book.

CHAPTER TWENTY FOUR
PHASE III WEIGHT TRAINING

As we have found, the key to making gains in the gym is not an exercise, or group of exercises, or number of reps. It is finding the right frequency, volume and intensity that will allow you to gradually improve. Finding the right combination that when you consistently overload over the course of time, you build strength and muscle.

The base workouts in Phase I are awesome. But let's say you have some lagging body parts. Remember way back when I talked about how stupid single joint exercises like dumbbell kick backs are? Well, I still think they are stupid for shaping, but they make great sense if you have a lagging body part.

After building up a base amount of muscle and then losing the fat, you can now see what your muscles really look like.

I had always thought I had big pecs. And I did. But once I got the fat off I realized I had no upper chest. All those years of dips, what a waste.

So, I toyed around with a workouts and wound up with a couple different versions in the same pattern. I'll give you the pattern first.

Monday
AM Sprints
PM Weights

Tuesday
AM Sprints
PM Weights

Wednesday
AM Nothing
PM Weights

Thursday
Off or functional distance

Friday
AM Sprints

PM Weights

Saturday
AM Easy Intervals, Agility or Nothing
PM Weights

Sunday—Off

I will throw in a little caveat, I don't do cardio the day after I train legs. I have a whole section on cardio later in the book. It is a complicated subject.

The pattern above is one I really like. It works well for me. Will it work well for you? I don't know.

If you are not into experimentation, stick with what you know works—the basic workouts from Phase I. They just about always work and are easy to adjust in terms of volume, frequency, and intensity.

When I get back from a few months in a war zone, I always start back with a basic Phase I approach—build back the muscle I lost from living in the dirt.

Here is the workout I am doing right now. This is really only for a Phase III guy who has already spent a month or more on the base workout and is looking for something different.

Monday
AM Sprints
PM Standing Dumbbell Shoulder Press 3 sets
        Machine Lateral Raises 3 sets
        Leaning Single Arm Side Laterals 2 sets

Tuesday
AM Sprints
PM Hack Squat 2 sets
        Lying Leg Curls 2 sets
        Toe risers 2 sets

Wednesday
AM Nothing
PM Wide Grip Lat Pull downs 3 sets

Machine Row 3 sets
Machine Rear Delt Flys 2 sets
Smith Machine Shrugs 2 sets

Thursday - Off

Friday
AM Sprints
PM Barbell Flat Bench Press 3 sets
Machine Incline 3 sets

Saturday
AM Easy Interval Running and/or Agility
PM Tricep Extensions 3 sets
Barbell Curls 3 sets
Skull Crushers, wide grip 3 sets
Dumbbell Curls 2 sets each arm

Sunday—Off

I still take each set to failure and depending on where I am in my pre-expedition training I take from 25 to eight breaths between sets. These days I only count my first set toward my magic number. When I get to 10 reps on the first set, I increase the weight the next week.

These workouts only take 10-20 minutes, tops. But, at the end of each workout I know I've worked out.

I don't lollygag around between exercises. I move fast when racking up my weight. Some people comment that I, "really don't do very much in the gym." As you should understand by now, I am doing what works for me.

As for the weights I'm moving, I am not absurdly strong, but stronger than I will ever need to be for Iraq. I recently barbell bench pressed 315 pounds for ten reps. I am up to 270 pounds for lat pull downs. A few weeks ago I was doing dumbbell rows with 150 pounds.

These days I tend to finish off with what I call a 'flail' as in 'flailing about'. For barbell curls say I got ten solid reps, clean, no crazy jerk or swing. But, when I went for 11, I could only move it a few inches. So I will stand there for a bit, just trying to move it that few inches a few times. No jerking, no swinging, not even 'flailing' really. If I do that I will note it in the log book as '10 + flail'.

Sometimes I'm able to get a half of a rep. So I will note that as '10.5' in the log book. Which leads to the occasional '10.5 + flail' entry in the log book. For tracking purposes I only increase the weight when I hit my magic number with clean reps.

What I have found after years of following the principle of overload over time is that max overload works for me. When I mean every set to failure every time, I mean absolute crushing failure to where I even spend time trying to move a weight I cannot move. This level of intense failure may be too much for a lot of people.

Now here is a strange thing about me. I rarely ever train with a partner so I try to avoid exercises where I need a spotter. I don't do forced reps, where you have a spotter help you get the last few reps, I don't do negatives. I will do drop sets on occasion, but am not doing them now.

I have nothing against forced reps, but they are hard to track. How much weight was your spotter moving versus your effort? A guess at best. This is not to argue against doing forced reps and negatives. In fact, if you have a competent training partner, I would suggest a 'fourth set'.

The 'fourth set' is not really a stand alone set, just a way of counting forced reps. When you are at the end of the third set and you can no longer perform clean reps, your spotter can help you with forced reps or negatives.

For tracking purposes only the clean reps count toward the magic number. The forced reps or negatives, even though you never rack the weight are the "fourth set".

The tabulation for tracking purposes would like this:

> *Barbell Shoulder Press*
> 185 x 9 1st Set
>   x 5 2nd Set
>   x 2 3rd Set
>   x 5 Forced Reps 4th Set
>   Total 16

After the two clean reps in the third set, your training partner would help you do as many more as you could, but these forced reps would be counted as the 'fourth set'. How do you know if you've done enough forced reps? That is actually determined by your partner. On an exercise like shoulder press, if your partner is lifting more than 20% of the load, it is probably time to rack the weight. The key to forced reps and negatives is a competent spotter. A person you can trust to get it right. There are rarely random people at the gym I trust to get it right. I don't have a regular workout partner, so, at this stage, I do not do them.

One of the other things you will notice is that I'm still not doing very many exercises. Even after all these years, my volume is still pretty low. For me, at this stage, I think I'm doing the maximum number of exercises/sets I could do. The five day rotation outlined above works for me. Will it work for you? Maybe. Who knows. Give it a shot, track your results. If it works, stick with it. If it doesn't, end the experiment and go back to what you know works.

That is the purpose of tracking. That is why I harp on it so much, nag you about it so much. If you are tracking your progress, you will be able to determine what works for you.

For my diet, I eat the same thing Sunday through Friday. I weigh everything. If I'm gonna be working on set, filming something or in the studio or on the road, I try to pack as much of my own food as possible.

What works for me is cooking a bunch of steak ahead of time. I weigh it out, put it in re-sealable bowls, throw in some broccoli and freeze it. I get a lot of my cooking done on Sunday. Then all I have to do is toss a bowl in the microwave and few minutes later my steak is done. If I'm gonna be on the road that day, I toss a few steak meals in the cooler.

Every convenience store has a microwave. I buy a bottle of water, cook my frozen steak meal and I'm still on the eating plan. I'll put some whey powder in a shaker and then all I have to do is add water for a quick snack.

If I'm gonna be traveling out of town, that can be a serious pain. I try to stay in an extended-stay hotel that has a little kitchenette. I'll bring my oats with me and whey powder. Then I hit a grocery store, buy some steak and eggs and bam, I'm still on the plan or close enough to it.

I do train out of town when I can. If I can get into a gym, I will get some lifting in. If I can't get into a gym, I can still do some cardio. But I have found that if I try to really train hard while living in a hotel and spending a full day behind the camera, I get run down.

My rule—do a little something physical, try to stay close to the eating plan.

Phase III is forever. If you fall off the wagon for a few days, whatever. You know how to get back on.

If I'm in the United States during football season, that tends to kill me. I'm either part of a TV crew working the game or, I'm doing what I really love to do—eat and watch football. If I'm part of the crew, I pack my food and do well. But if I am not part of a TV crew, I turn into mega couch potato fan. There is nothing like a pizza and watching the prime-time Saturday night college football game. Followed by doughnuts and pastries while watching the Sunday pre-game shows. To top it off, brats on a bun and salty, carby snacks during six hours of football games.

Of course, we know the consequences of that pigskin bliss. If I start to put on fat, the solution is easy-cut out Sunday afternoon and/or Sunday morning.

Cheating is fine, if you understand the results of going off the plan. And since we now understand it, we can control it, adapt it, modify it.

If my girlfriend wants to go out on a Thursday night to one of my favorite Mexican restaurants, I may go ahead and have all the chips and carbs I want. But on Saturday, I will tame back the cheat to a controlled refeed of just some extra oatmeal or just a large green salad. The refeed concept will be addressed in the following chapter.

Refeeds and resets have an important role. In many ways, Phase III is all about resets.

CHAPTER TWENTY FIVE
TRICKING YOUR METABOLISM

"Improvise, adapt, overcome," was Clint Eastwood's line in the movie Heartbreak Ridge. As a Marine, that line is etched in my consciousness. When faced with an obstacle, improvise, adapt, overcome.

Your body, will also improvise, adapt and attempt to overcome whatever you throw at it as well. It will try to find homeostasis and adapt to the 'new normal'. Your body likes to plateau. Nothing is more frustrating than getting stuck, hitting the plateau, not making any progress.

I got stuck in building muscle and tried to break through, but it never worked. It didn't work because I was not using systematic overload that prevented adaptation by the muscles. In losing fat, you will run into the opposite of this problem. You can only go so low on the calories. You can only get to near zero on the carbs and sugars.

There is not a way to systematically, over the course of months and months, to keep reducing calories, sugars and carbs. Eventually you get to a level that cannot be sustained, or, if you find a sustainable level, your body will adapt to it, adjusting your metabolism at that level.

Since I am not looking to compete in a bodybuilding contest, the goal for me is maintenance and the occasional slow, steady stretch of fat loss.

Carb cycling is a tool kit solution. It only works in bursts. It is not much of a lifestyle. I found the solution to prevent my body from adapting in doing something very simple and enjoyable—pigging out. But we'll call it something fancy like metabolic reset.

Once you have worked your way backwards through your meals, cut out the sugars, cut out the carbs and have found the diet that allows you to lose fat while being able to get through the work day, eventually, your body will adapt to it.

You will stop losing fat.

I used to get so frustrated and say to myself, "I'll never have abs," and drone on through workouts saying that it was okay to be in way better shape than most guys my age.

And it is. If that is your goal, use the weight lifting techniques in Phase I and principles of this system to build muscle and strength and enjoy being big and strong! Nothing wrong with being heavy duty—unless you do not want to be heavy duty.

For a while I was convinced I would always be a heavy duty guy.

But when I started really working on losing fat, I applied the same kind of tracking and it started taking fat off. A systematic underload overtime. The ketogenic carb cycles being the logical conclusion of that underload.

But, there is still the plateau.

Applying the systematic overload line of reasoning to my diet, I realized that I just needed to change up. Just like when I tell you to quit doing military press when you can no longer increase the number of reps or amount of weight, when you quit losing fat, and can't cut out any more sugar or carbs, it is time to change up.

This change up is the metabolic reset, or pigging out.

But before we go into pigging out and the way to do it effectively, lets hone in on tracking again.

You need four tools to track body composition:

1. Your training log book
2. A scale
3. A pair of body fat calipers
4. A cloth tape measure.

As you may have noticed, I recommend these tools often.

Your log book will tell you if you are getting stronger, or weaker, or staying the same. There is a muscle memory effect to some exercises—the more often you do them, the more effective your body is at firing all the muscles in sequence. But, as a general rule, if you are getting stronger over time, you are building muscle. If you are holding steady, your are maintaining your muscle. If you are getting weaker you are losing muscle.

But, to dial in on whether you are building muscle or maintaining muscle, you need to use a quantifiable measure like lean tissue diameter.

The scale is a crude instrument at best, but it has its place. The key is to weigh yourself at the same time of day. If your eating is consistent, then that variable is taken away and the trend will be accurate. A rule statisticians follow is that even a flawed measurement, over time, shows the trend accurately.

For the scale, what counts is the number over time—as in weeks not days.

Third is the cheap body fat calipers. A thirty dollar set is just fine. Our goal with the calipers is not to measure percentage of body fat, very few experts can do that effectively. Ours is a very simple measurement, millimeters of thickness on the lower outside abs where the rectus abdominals meet the obliques. Just like with the scale, do it at the same time, the same way, on the same side so even if the measurement itself is flawed, the trend is accurate. Only bother to check the millimeters of thickness once a week.

And of course, write down your weight and millimeters of thickness and lean tissue diameter measurements in your training book so you can track your progress, or lack of, overtime.

In the weight training, following the principle of overload over time, what should you do if you plateau on the number of reps for any exercise? That's right, quit doing it and start doing a new one that works the same bodypart(s).

But now we are going to be tracking body composition using the quantifiable measures above. Looking at yourself in the mirror is not a quantifiable measurement. Progress photos don't lie, but are hard to control the variables—light, distance from the lens, holding the exact same pose, even what you are wearing can throw it off.

But the three crude instruments—scale, calipers, tape measure have hard statistical numbers, just like the amount of weight you move for a given number of reps. Here are the questions you need to answer as you continue toward your goals:

- Is your weight trending up, down or holding even?
- Is your strength moving up, down or holding even?
- Are the millimeters of fat thickness going up, down or holding even?
- Is the lean tissue diameter increasing, decreasing or staying the same?

Guessing doesn't work. Tracking works.

If you are trying to cut fat, the key measure is obviously millimeters of fat thickness and lean muscle diameter.

If you are trying to build muscle, lean tissue diameter and weight are what want to watch.

If you are trying to maintain, obviously you just want everything to be static.

Eventually though, your body's metabolism will adjust, especially if you cease to put on muscle. To break through that metabolic plateau, you may need to reset your metabolism.

Here is a metabolic reset that has worked for me:

> 1. Stop all cardio. Barely lift weights in the gym. Increase carbs by 100 percent. Do this for a week.

> 2. Have two full on crazy, eat everything in sight cheat days on the last two days of the reset.

Your body will freak out. It will not know what to do, but it will decide that this is the new normal and adapt to it.

Then you go back to what we did before, gradually cut back on the carbs, start doing cardio again and gradually increase the duration and intensity.

And the cheat day or cheat meal?

You bet. Have it. Go crazy. But still incorporate it into the system and it gradually goes from a crazy all day frenzy of beer, pizza and cupcakes to just having an extra bowl of oatmeal on Saturday.

Like the systematic overload in the gym, your goal is to hit a lower number of millimeters every time you plateau.

Remember the example of Rob, who by looking in his training logs could tell you where he plateaued at doing incline bench over the course of years and how each time the plateau was a few pounds heavier?

Well, our goal is that every time you plateau on your diet, where you can't go any lower on the carbs, sugars, the millimeters of fat as measured by the same calipers are smaller—or at least never going up.

Do a reset and start over again. Underload over time.

You know by now why the overload over time principle works: The muscles are constantly forced to adapt to a constantly progressing overload.

The body will also adapt to any eating plan. You can only underload calories for a few weeks before the body hits a plateau. Your body will even adapt to ketosis. Your metabolic rate will find a balance.

The only solution I have found is metabolic reset. I just made up the term 'metabolic reset'. It is just a fancy way to say take a week off and eat more, but what it does is throw off the pathways of what is called the Krebs cycle.

The Krebs cycle, named after Hans Krebs, is the cycle by which food is turned into energy. In other words, metabolism. The cycle is sensitive to the intake of food and demands on output of energy.

Just like in the ketogenic carb cycle, where the body is tricked into burning nothing but fat by going to no carbs, then loading up on carbs, then going back to no carbs, the metabolic reset is all about messing with Krebs cycle.

The Saturday cheat is the same thing, but on a smaller scale.

Your body will try to bring everything into alignment. It will adapt to an underload of calories and carbs and an increase in exercise like cardio. Gradually building muscle prevents the body from adapting as the increased muscle burns more calories.

But, by this stage, the muscle gains are slow and the body will slowly adapt.

The Saturday cheat throws the body and Krebs cycle out of whack for a few hours. It has to work at processing all that sugar, carbs and fat it normally doesn't get. Usually, the Saturday insanity is enough to keep the metabolism from adapting to your eating and exercise. But eventually, it will catch up to you.

When that happens, it is time for a metabolic reset, or, taking time off from the gym and eating more.

One of my typical metabolic resets begins on a Thursday.

Normally I may do some functional distance running on Thursday, but during reset, I say screw the running. I also throw in an extra big bowl of oatmeal and maybe eat out at an Italian restaurant getting plenty of pasta and bread. I still eat all my protein.

I don't train at all on Friday and eat like I did on Thursday.

Saturday, still no training and I go crazy. I still try to get close to all my protein, but will go on a marathon of carbs, sugar, fat. Anything that strikes my fancy.

Sunday, same as Saturday, but I get back on the base eating plan in the evening.

I typically start to feel like crap on Sunday afternoon. My body is all freaked out. I'm bloated, holding water and probably 10 pounds heavier—or more than I was on Wednesday.

On Monday, I am strong and by Tuesday, I feel like a fat burning furnace.

Another metabolic reset I use that is less fun, but more effective, is to just not train for a week. Let the muscles heal up and soak up nutrients. Stick close to the base diet, maybe add in some more oats and let your body adapt to doing less exercise.

Since Phase III is forever, taking time off is not a big deal. I know what will happen, and if I do it when my body needs it, it allows me to continue to make gradual gains.

I do some type of reset every couple months. Of course for me, the ultimate reset is a three month trip to Iraq to film a documentary or TV show.

What do I do when I've been off the wagon for three months? What should you do if you've fallen off the wagon for a few months? Start over at Phase I.

It is inevitable. Life will get in the way. You will get a new job, or start up a business, or take on a huge project, have a baby. I cannot imagine going for 30 years nonstop. Life just won't let it happen.

When life happens to me, like shooting for three months in Afghanistan, I do what I can to stay in shape while there. Eat the best I can, do what I can to train. But at times I am just living in the dirt in the middle of a war. Which is why I train so hard using this system before I find myself living in the dirt in the middle of a war.

We all know what that guy would do if life got in the way. Since you are no longer that guy, get back into Phase I, run the system again. And you know what, because you understand it so well, because you know what works specifically for you, you will rebound freakishly fast.

As fun as planned metabolic resets and the weekend cheat can be, there is a more effective method to keep the metabolism off balance that harnesses the power of mathematics. This method could be expressed as:

$$X_{n+1} = (aX_n + b) \bmod m$$

which is an algorithm used to generate a string of random numbers.

Or, the coin flip eating plan.

CHAPTER TWENTY SIX
RANDOM EATING

The body will always try to adapt to what it detects as the new normal or a trend to the new normal. In the weight room, overload over time works because the new normal is always a heavier weight or more reps and muscles are always adapting upward. In the kitchen, when carbs and sugars are progressively cut back, the body adjusts the metabolism downward. The underload works to lose fat when the carbs/sugars/calories are cut faster than the body can adapt.

But what if we want to stretch the underload out even longer until the body adapts? How could we trick the body into never adapting to a normal during a slow, gradual underload? By flipping a coin. Or, more precisely, harnessing the underlying randomness of a coin toss.

Randomness is a powerful mathematical and analytical tool. Surveys and opinion polls use a randomly selected sample of people to accurately gauge the mood of the whole. In medical trials, randomization is used to determine who gets the placebo and who gets the treatment being tested. In medical randomization, if the group of people in the subject population pool is large enough, then the variables will be equal in the group receiving the placebo or the actual treatment.

The Random Walk Hypothesis is used by economists and investors to determine if the rise in value of a stock is merely haphazard or an actual trend. Randomness is also used to determine if there really is a pattern or trend in the earnings of a company.

Take a look at this chart showing the earnings of a company:

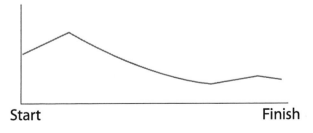

Start   Finish

Is the stock a good buy, or a loser? Has it bottomed out and is ready to make a come-back? Is the CEO a moron? Given that I created the data points by flipping a coin 10 times, who knows.

I started with the arbitrary number 50 and flipped a quarter. If it was heads, the 'earnings' went up 20 percent. If was tails, it went down 20 percent. The small run of coming up heads at the end meant the 20 percent was only a 20 percent increase in earnings from the very bottom.

What looks like a trend, the drop in 'earnings' was just a random string of the coin toss coming up tails. A random string of the coin toss coming up heads could make the CEO of the company look like a genius.

If our brain can be fooled into a seeing a trend in randomness—the body can be tricked even easier because all the body knows is what is happening now and what happened for the past few days.

Randomness can also be applied to the eating plan to keep the body from ever finding the new normal and adjusting the metabolism and in reality, it doesn't even need to be random. Luckily for us the body does not collect and analyze data using regression analysis or else it would figure out what we were doing really fast and refuse to be gamed any longer.

Just like the weekly pig out or weekly metabolic reset is used to keep the body off balance, a random variation in carbohydrate intake, which also affects to total caloric intake can be used to keep the metabolism from ever truly adapting. If carbohydrate intake is varied randomly, the body can never adjust to the new normal.

To do this is as simple as flipping a coin. Heads means that day the base diet is eaten. Tails means 50 percent less carbohydrates are eaten. If the base diet is 100 grams of carbs, a tails day means only 50 grams of carbs are eaten.

If charted, the random walk may look something like this:

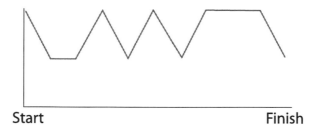

Start   Finish

A coin flip is random over the course of many flips. There will be strings where heads comes up five time in a row, but over the course of time it equals out. If heads keeps coming up, impose a little short term variation by having a low carb day.

On the higher carb days the metabolism will want to speed up a little bit, on the low carb days the metabolism will still be higher creating a short term underload. No adaptation can truly be made.

This randomness can also be used while dieting to lose fat.

If the base diet is 100 grams of carbs per day, in the first week, alternate between 20 percent fewer carbs and 50 percent fewer carbs. Heads means 80 grams of carbs. Tails means 50 grams of carbs.

The following week the base is number is now 80 grams of carbs. Heads would be 64 grams of carbs (80 x .20 = 16,   80 – 16 = 64). Tails would mean 40 grams of carbs.

Here is what a random walk down in carbs might look like over time:

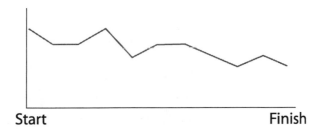

Start   **Finish**

Applying randomness to a systematic underload of carbohydrates gives the body two things to try and adapt to—the overall reduction in carbs and the random variation between carbohydrate intake on a daily basis. The Krebs cycle will never be able to adapt in time. You will always be ahead of the cycle.

The body will try to seek balance and adapt to the new normal. This adaptation process is used to great advantage in adding muscle and can be manipulated in eating through metabolic resets or randomness.

Where the body's ability to adapt will really come in to play is with cardio.

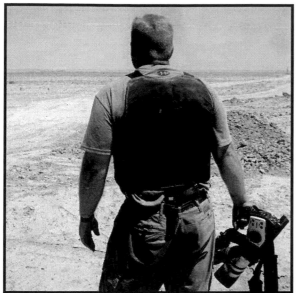

Left: North of Kharmah, Iraq, Summer 2005.

With CPL John Hegland, the day after our crazy roof run.

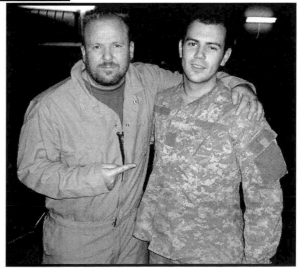

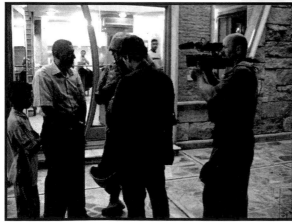

Left: Filming in the Saidiya district of Baghdad, October 2008.

Right: With the Khalidiyah Police, Spring 2007.

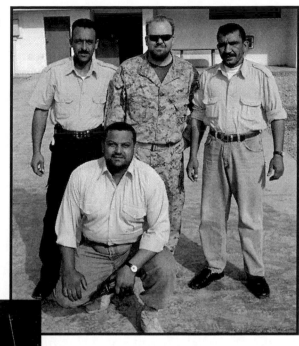

After a workout with Nita, Winter 2009.

Right: With General Ray Odierno after filming an interview for TIME.

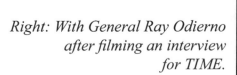

——————— CHAPTER TWENTY SEVEN ———————
THE CARDIO DILEMMA

Cardio will make you gain fat. Cardio can help you lose fat.

Those statements seem mutually exclusive, but they are not.

Bodybuilders don't run. I'm not a bodybuilder. But after Phase III, a lot of you are looking like one.

This is a subject I wrestle with. For me, cardio is a necessity. I need speed, stamina and endurance to survive in Iraq and Afghanistan. I have to be 'Fit for Combat'. I need to pack the most punch in the most efficient package.

And this is where you need to make an informed, personal decision. I think the cardio system I have worked out to make me 'Fit for Combat' will be great for nearly everyone. Especially if you want some functional cardio/athletic performance. If you want to do what I do—great. But make an informed decision.

Lisa and Glen Krog, my friends from South Africa, are great trainers. As I wrote way back in Part I, they say "no cardio". Lisa stays super lean year round and does not do cardio. Glen competes in bodybuilding contests and never does cardio.

Nita, does cardio. As a fitness competitor, she needs the conditioning to perform her routine. She does sprints, middle distance, plyometrics, stadium stairs, intervals. Nita carries a lot of muscle, is really lean and does a lot of cardio. The track work and intervals are a part of the training program for nearly every competitor Nita trains.

So, who is right? Is cardio good or bad?

Here we have three undeniable experts. People who compete at the top of level of the muscle game and train clients to get on stage. Yet, they disagree on cardio. Or do they?

Actually, they do not disagree on one key. It is fundamental principle, your body will adapt to cardio and there will be diminishing returns. Just like how the body will adapt to changes in diet and overload over time with the weights, the body will adapt to cardio work with some negative effects.

Remember how Lisa explained it back in Chapter 16:

> "If the energy in, energy out formula worked, you would be able to cardio yourself out of existence.
>
> "If you did enough cardio every day to burn 500 more calories than you ate, after a few years you would simply not exist. But all those people putting in hours on the cardio machines for years still exist."

Cardio vascular exercise also has some negative effects on muscle mass. Lisa and Glen explain them below:

> First, cardiovascular activity is very efficient at chewing up muscle tissue, the steps are as follows:
>
> 1. Conversion from fast twitch muscle fiber to slow twitch muscle fiber, by acquiring mitochondria and relinquishing contractile protein. Smaller fiber, less RMR.
>
> 2. Excessive Cortisol released in response to the damage to the fiber as a result of the exercise. Cortisol acts as a natural analgesic, but severely hampers protein synthesis and muscle repair. It also damages the immune system, and ultimately will contribute to all of our deaths - so I'm not sure why anyone would do anything that would accelerate this process.
>
> 3. It has been shown, that high volume cardiovascular exercise can completely deplete satellite cells in muscle fiber, which means no new fiber can grow or existing fiber be repaired.
>
> 4. Growth Hormone levels decline with high volume cardiovascular exercise, which also hampers the repair process. Low growth hormone also accelerates aging.
>
> 5. To sum it up, you can't train all day, and you can't eat no food, but you can always build a bit more muscle, so quit the cardio and concentrate on the weight lifting.

Cardio can make you fat and less muscular and that my friends is one hell of an argument for never doing cardio. If your goal is appearance oriented and you don't have to be 'Fit for Combat' Lisa and Glen will tell you to stop doing cardio. Over the long haul, lifting hard and a controlled eating plan will give you a better looking physique.

Okay, but what about the short term? Is cardio useful in burning off fat when you use it in conjunction with weight training and a controlled eating plan?

Cardio is best done as part of a plan to achieve a goal. It is a tool. A way to get from point A to point B in your fitness goals. When I was really working on taking the fat off I did a lot of old-fashioned long term cardio. I gradually increased the duration and intensity over the course of months. The cardio, combined with a controlled eating plan, did its job to a certain point. Then it essentially quit working. I think the only reason it worked as long as it did was because I had previously built up so much muscle.

When the long duration cardio, 45 minutes in the

NITA SPEAKS

With high-intensity interval training you can go for less time, more intensity (in spurts) and stay consistent in your body's abilities to use fat for fuel, which is what everyone wants.

With high-intensity interval training you "sprint" on any cardio exercise for short bursts that go for less than two minutes, and then you slow to moderate, and sometimes even low-intensity pace for a short burst. You want to go high intensity to kick your heart rate way up, and then you drop the intensity to less your body rest, while not giving your heart rate enough time to drop out beneath a fat-burning zone. If you do this for short bursts of time, you don't give your heart rate a chance to drop severely, and therein, you are able to keep your body burning fat, burning calories, and staying hard at work, even though you won't feel like you're working hard while your body recovers during your lower-paced durations.

Like cardio, this too can strengthen your heart, and keep you from feeling sluggish. On the other hand, in comparison to cardio, interval training burns fat for longer periods of time. You will burn fat for up to 13 hours post-workout with intervals, whereas with cardio at a constant moderate rate will only burn fat efficiently for up to 2 hours post workout. So, why would you spend more time and burn less fat, much less want to gamble the possibility of kicking out cortisol? This is why many fitness professionals who know what they are doing will not recommend long dull high, low or medium-intensity periods of cardio.

morning and 30 minutes before lifting weights quit working, I didn't just pile on more cardio. I did a metabolic reset, hit the weights harder, kept my eating on track and took Nita's advise and started running sprints.

When I started running sprints, I was able to lose fat without really trying that hard. Sometimes, doing less is more effective than doing more.

I often see people in the gym who have kept doing so much more, kept adding so much more cardio, that it is difficult for them to make any progress. Excessive cardio done on a regular basis prevents more people from reaching their goals than you would ever imagine, last summer, it happened to a friend of mine.

My friend Natasha is an exercising machine. I've done workouts with her and they kick my ass. She was a gymnast and ballerina in her youth—a well rounded athlete. She's in her late twenties, has a son and a gorgeous body. She has a great career as an accountant and during tax season life happens and she gains a few pounds, but during the Summer she gets back in the gym, doing her totally bad ass workouts and gets her great body back.

Natasha is not as muscular as Nita and never gets nearly as lean as Lisa. She likes to keep her curves—but with a tightness and shape from muscle.

Natasha decided she wanted to get a little leaner and build up some more muscle. Her workouts were insane—volume on the level of the 'Armageddon Arm Workout'. She will do a set of bench press, then jump rope for 60 seconds then do another set of bench. Then on top of that she did even more cardio! Her diet was already well controlled and as an accountant, she needs serious brain power all day long.

The solution could not be to add more cardio—she was already super fit cardiovascular wise. Diet wasn't much of an option. And she already lifted a lot of weights. How do you take someone at that level of fitness, with a great body and jump them to the next level?

Well, that is similar to the whole dilemma we face with cardio. If you are heavy duty or extra chubbisome at Phase II, increased cardio—increasing your cardio load over time will help you lose the fat.

But what happens when you reach your goal. You are lean and it is time to get on to Phase III? If you cut the cardio cold turkey, you will have, at least on paper, a calorie surplus. Calorie surpluses tend to become fat.

All that cardio that got you lean will now come back to haunt you.

Even worse, all the cardio plus the low carb or ketosis. A double down on a caloric surplus.

This is the classic dieters rebound that Atkins dieters experience the worst. They stop the diet, go back to eating carbs and sugar and blow up like balloons.

What was the solution for Natasha? There was no way to create even more of a deficit through exercise. Diet was not an option and she was damned if she was gonna do an intentional rebound—even if I called something fancy like a 'metabolic reset'.

The solution for Natasha was a 'walk back' or controlled exercise underload. All that cardio and training volume was never going to allow her to build more muscle. But a rapid decline in exercise output would cause a calorie surplus.

She took up my five day rotation from Phase III, quit doing the jump rope between sets but still did the regular cardio. In the first weeks something interesting happened—she got stronger. All those calories and nutrients that were being burned up in her super set 'Armageddon' workouts were redirected toward the muscle repair.

Natasha underloaded the cardio, gradually decreasing the duration and intensity.

As she did that, she discovered she could put more intensity into every set of weight training.

The process took six weeks. In her particular situation she was then able to start substituting carbs and the few sugars she was eating with protein. Once all the cardio was gone and 'Armageddon' workouts brought down to reality, she found she didn't need all the carbs. She got leaner and her muscles—which were being starved and burned from all the cardio—filled out.

The key to cardio is knowing its place. Overload over time is something you do forever with the weights. The controlled eating with metabolic resets and randomization tricks is something you can do forever. Cardio is something you keep in the tool kit for when you need it.

Most people will need it during Phase I and Phase II. And I think I have come up with a really good open architecture system to find a cardio plan that works for you.

—————————— **CHAPTER TWENTY EIGHT** ——————————
SPRINTS

The cardio system I use now is one anyone can keep in their toolkit to use when they need it.

It is good for beginners and the open architecture allows it to be used for people with an intermediate level or advanced level of fitness.

The majority of my cardio conditioning for my work in combat zones is sprints. I still do some functional distance work, but it is purely functional.

Here is my sprinting/cardio rotation, I'll get into duration and distance in a moment:

Monday AM
Sprints

Tuesday AM
Sprints

Wednesday AM
None

Thursday AM
None/or Functional Distance

Friday AM
Sprints

Saturday AM
None/or Easy Interval/or Agility Drills

Sunday AM—None

I like sprinting as the foundation because there is an open architecture to sprints. Sprints also keep the metabolism elevated longer and are just close enough to weight lifting that they don't lead to muscle catabolism.

With distance work or normal cardio the only variables are time, duration, speed, and intensity.

With sprints you can alter:
>   Duration/Distance of Sprint
>   Duration of workout
>   Duration of recovery between sprints
>   Intensity/speed

One of my favorite sprinting workouts is what I call the "Flying 50," as in 50 yards. I do my sprints on a football field. Nita does hers on a college running track. A person could even use a parking lot or a long flat stretch of road.

The flying fifty uses the length of the field—100 yards from goal line to goal line Starting at the goal line, sprint to the 50 yard line.

Decelerate, which will take 10-20 yards, walk the remaining 30-40 yards to the goal line.

Turn around.

Sprint to the 50 yard line.

Decelerate, which will take 10-20 yards, walk the remaining 30-40 yards to the goal line.

Turn around.

Sprint to the 50 yard line.

You are seeing the pattern.

If you have not been doing any running or sprinting, do not try to sprint all out on your first time doing this workout. Jogging it the first time is just fine. Work your way up to where you do a few "Flying 50s" at a good stride. Then try to sprint it.

What I do is pick a number of minutes. When I first started doing the "Flying 50s" I was already running a lot, so I picked ten minutes. I try to get as many repetitions as I can in ten minutes. You may want to start at three or four minutes. (Or you could pick a number of repetitions and try to get them done as quickly as possible.)

When you get to a point that you just can't get any more repetitions in the determined number of minutes, increase the duration of the workout by a minute or two.

Hey, doesn't this sound just like overload overtime? Indeed it is.

What if the "Flying 50" sounds a little too intense? No problem. Try "Looped 50s."

Start at the goal line.

Sprint to the 50 yard line.

Decelerate to a walk. Turnaround and walk back to the goal line you started at. Turn around and sprint to the 50 yard line again.

The "Looped 50" gives you a longer break between sprints.

Manage your overload over time the same way. Try to get as many repetitions as you can in a set number of minutes. When you plateau, add a minute or two to the duration of the workout.

Sprints allow you to vary so many things. You can do 75 yards, 100 yards. You can make your recovery between sprints based on time, distance walked or decline in heart rate.

If you have a friend who will help you, then the actual elapsed time of the sprints can be something you use as part of your overload over time. Your first few sprints will always be pretty fast, but the later ones, especially when you get to 100 yards, will be slower, so you can try to beat a certain time in the later sprints or track it through average elapsed time.

I use sprints as the foundation of my cardio conditioning to be able to work in Iraq and Afghanistan. Therefore, I am always doing them or some type of cardio conditioning. You may not want or need that kind of conditioning. You may need it just as a tool to get some fat off, and sprints are great at taking the fat off.

The rest of my cardio conditioning to be 'Fit for Combat" is pretty easy. Once a week I do some functional distance—two miles. I try to keep improving the time, but am not as intense about it as I am at tracking the overload overtime with the sprints.

On Saturday I may or may not do some easy intervals. I do the easy intervals around the neighborhood. I walk for a block, run for a block (not jog, run), walk, run, walk, run, for a few minutes longer than the duration of my sprints. I will mix in some agility drills and plyometrics on Saturdays as well.

There are a lot of varying ideas on when you should do cardio. Some people are adamant about doing it first thing in the morning, before breakfast. Others will say before you lift weights. Others after lifting weights. A few will even say before bed time.

NITA SPEAKS

Sprints are high intensity bursts of energy which optimize muscle usage in going beyond the slow twitch fibers most used in our legs into the fast twitch fibers, which ultimately develops muscle. Muscular development increases fat burning because more muscle causes increased metabolism.

In addition, short bursts of energy optimize caloric burn. If you are looking to increase conditioning, fat burning and caloric optimization and efficiency, then short burst of energy like sprints are really the only alternative. In short, sprints are a quicker path to leanness than most any cardio.

I do my sprints right after I wake up. I stumble into the kitchen, have some whey with water, glutamine and amino tabs, put on my running shoes and walk 400 yards to the football field, stretch a bit then dive in.

I like doing sprints in the morning because then they are out of the way. They help wake me up and energize my mind before I sit down to edit video or write a script.

With this cardiovascular conditioning program I have struck a balance between muscle/strength/power and speed/stamina/endurance that is similar to combat.

Combat operations often last for hours upon hours and require only a moderate level of output—walking with all your gear on. In some environments it is a lot of walking, vaulting over walls, climbing buildings, jumping rooftops.

But at any moment things can get really intense. Combat goes from five miles per hour to 100 in a split second. And the benefit of being 'Fit for Combat' is not all about being able to keep up with that speed.

The real combat benefit is in motor coordination and mental clarity.

As your heart rate goes up, it is harder to do manual tasks. It is harder to think clearly, to focus. Obviously, when the bullets are flying adrenaline is released, your heart rate will go up. But, if the increase of the rate from just the physical exertion is minimized through training—then it will be easier to do manual tasks and think clearly.

For a Paratrooper or Marine, the tasks are aiming, reloading, observation, fires coordination, using a radio or clearing a jammed weapon.

For me it is holding the camera steady, framing the shot and getting it in focus.

If you want to try something, sprint 100 yards all out then immediately try to take a picture with a digital camera or use your cell phone. Not that easy is it—and no one is trying to kill you on the football field!

Like I said way back at the beginning, for me fitness is a matter of life and death. If I can't think clearly in a fire fight, I put not only myself at risk but the lives of the Paratroopers and Marines I am with.

Which is why I am so intense about being 'Fit for Combat'.

PART III

THE ROAD FORWARD

CHAPTER TWENTY NINE
PERSONAL TRAINERS

So what happens next? For a lot of you, if you stick with a permanent Phase III or do Phase I again smartly, you will achieve your goals. If you stick with the principles—overload over time, tracking, accountability, controlled eating, metabolic resets, the coin flip eating plan and tool-kit cardio you will be able to gradually look better and better every year. You will gradually become stronger. You will be able to get back on the system after life happens.

What I hope I have shown you here is that there is no silver bullet. There is no perfect workout, there is no perfect diet. There is just a way to find the workout and diet that works perfectly for you and how to adjust it as your body and lifestyle changes.

A few of you will want to go beyond what this system can reveal for you and what you can learn about what works for you. To do that you will need to work with a true professional.

In most major cities it is not hard to find a professional—a real trainer of competitive bodybuilders. In smaller cities, after reading this book, you have more knowledge than most of the trainers around.

One of the most interesting things is that you may not even need to live in a major city to find the professional that is right for you.

Nita trains people for contests all across the United States. Her website, www. fitnessdirectives.com was designed specifically to be able to train anyone with an internet connection.

Glen and Lisa live in South Africa, but train people in the United States through their website www.uniquephysique.co.za

I still check in with the Miami Muscle Girls when I want to shake things up a bit.

Just keep a few things in mind—not every bodybuilder, figure or fitness competitor is going to be a great trainer. Michael Jordan and Magic Johnson were great basketball players, but they were lousy coaches.

I have come to believe that women are just better at bodybuilding than men. When a woman decides she wants to be a bodybuilder, fitness or figure competitor, she doesn't screw around. If it doesn't work, she won't do it. Women are very results oriented and their approach to training guys, I have found, is very results oriented. Women understand that bodybuilding is visual, and with the exception of fitness competitors like Nita, it is 100 percent visual. It is all about how you look. Women are more appearance oriented than men and women bodybuilders train for appearance.

Moreover, if a woman has taken her physique to elite competition level, going against every piece of genetic encoding and societal pressure, doesn't it make sense they will be able to do the same with a guy?

If you have followed the Phases and stuck with Phase III and are thinking about taking to the next level—a professional trainer will love you. But a lot of trainers are morons which is why it is important to find a trainer that works with people at higher levels.

A lot of the best trainers run boutique gyms. They do not mill through ten clients a day in a mega gym—they have a small,

NITA SPEAKS

Finding a personal trainer is not as easy as going to the gym and picking out someone who has a certification. I have met a ratio of 20 to one of trainers who suck compared to those who are truly qualified out of pool of those who have certifications.

Personal trainers are supposed to motivate, instruct, and challenge you. If you are interviewing trainers (yes, interview them! You are hiring someone to work **FOR YOU**), there are three things to ask, and these are the bottom lines. This is your health and fitness, so you can never be too methodical in your approach to it. Don't undermine the value of this task.

Can this person motivate you and hold you accountable? Evaluate their rapport toward you as well as others if you can, and ask yourself if there is a chemistry with that person that will help you feel comfortable listening to the when they instruct and hold you accountable.

Does this person have real experience with real results? Check out testimonial photos and referrals from past clients. If they have helped other real people, then they can probably help you.

Is the person physically capable of doing what is necessary to help you? For instance, if you are a guy who is going to powerlift and gain mass, a 90 pound trainer probably won't be able to spot you well with support and keep you guarded during your lifting sessions.

Be realistic with who you are choosing, and try to stick with a trainer who is in generally good shape themselves so you know they can be in tune with you as you are developing.

often dumpy looking gym in an industrial park or dying strip mall. But, when you go inside you see men and women competitors.

The best trainers are not cheap. But since you have done so much on your own and know how to do it on your own through the system in this book, all they are doing is working with you to refine your methods and show you a few techniques. So while the unit price may be high, you will not have to pay it often.

CHAPTER THIRTY
NO MAGIC PILL

Supplements are not the answer. There are good supplements, there are useful supplements, but there is no solution in a pill or powder.

Back when I was that guy, I would try everything. I always kept thinking, "this is gonna work." And many of the supplements really do work, but only if you are eating enough quality food and following the principles of overload over time. If you are doing everything else right, they might help you recover a little faster or make up for a slight nutritional deficit.

Right now though, I don't buy a lot of stuff at the health food store. My supplement regime is pretty pedestrian.

- Whey Protein
- Amino Acid Tabs
- Glutamine
- Multi Vitamin
- Vitamin C
- Vitamin B6 & B12
- Calcium
- Flax Oil

To make sure I take my few supplements every day I invested five dollars in a pill planner box like senior citizens use. That way, every daily intake is sitting on my kitchen counter so I won't forget.

One of the things you have may noticed that is missing from my supplement regime is fat burners. Why? Easy, I don't use them.

Muscle is the ultimate fat burner with sprints being a distant second.

I did use fat burning products for a long time but all that happened was I got strung out on Ephedra/Mua Huang. I was seriously addicted and after using them for so long they really messed up my metabolism. When ephedra was banned and I couldn't get it anymore I ballooned up—and I was also able to build muscle again.

Fat burners, if you feel you must use them or really want to use them are a short-term tool at best. I'm not in this for anything on the short term. My advice—don't use them.

When I got away from a bunch of supplements and meal replacement drinks is when I really started making progress. Why have a meal replacement drink when you can have a real meal?

The only time I have a meal replacement is out of desperation—when I'm in an odd situation and didn't plan properly. More often than not, I will find a fast food restaurant, order the grilled NOT BREADED chicken sandwich, toss the bun and just eat the chicken breast, lettuce and tomato.

Food is better than any supplement.

NITA SPEAKS

Fat burners. Do they work? Yes, but not for a long term affect. They can be unsafe when they are abused, like all things.

Fat burners should be used with caution because of their effects on your heart. You don't want to get carried away using these, acting as if they are a vitamin supplement. If you have a short term goal like a class reunion or wedding or competition, they are great in these cases.

Don't mistake their usage to be long term, **EVER**.

Do not use your fat burners for more than six weeks consecutively, and I would recommend at least six weeks in between uses as well.

The only time I would really recommend a meal replacement drink is for a guy whose metabolism is incredibly fast and who has hard time putting on any muscle. For these guys—and they are rare—a meal replacement drink may be the best alternative to choking down 12 meals a day of whole food.

Meal replacement drinks are also handy for people whose jobs do not allow them to eat at their desk, or while driving a truck, or while on the job site. In those situations, the minute or two it takes to guzzle down a drink may be all that is available, so the drink becomes a necessity. Just avoid the ones loaded with sugar.

Supplements are just that, a supplement to real, whole basic foods. Sometimes basic food is boring but it works and is less expensive than the supplements.

CHAPTER THIRTY ONE
PALETTE PREPARATIONS

I have one pre-disposition that helps me.

I am not a genetically gifted bodybuilder or athlete. My metabolism has always been slow and I have horrible insulin reaction to carbs and sugar. I have a slightly above average ability to build muscle—I think. I'm really not sure though because I have always lifted weights.

But my real gift, if you want to call it a gift, is an unrefined palette. What food tastes like really doesn't matter to me. And when I really started controlling my eating I began to see food for what it is—fuel.

Now, I am still not the guy who can choke down dry boiled chicken or plain tuna out of the can. I like to have some taste. So I cook my strip steaks over natural wood charcoal. Natural wood charcoal and pepper make a great steak. I usually spend Sunday afternoon or evening cooking up several pounds of steak that I divide into containers and keep in the freezer ready to go.

Steak, though not the best protein, is very satisfying and has great flavor and texture even after being frozen and microwaved.

For breakfast I am an oatmeal guy. Or oatmeal, a vanilla flavored whey powder, flax oil, cinnamon and Splenda guy. Oatmeal was the only place I could find to hide the flax oil. I find flax oil repugnant. Some people can take it by the spoon. I need to cover it up with cinnamon and Splenda.

Eggs are a pretty plain food. They are probably the gold-standard of protein, but pretty bland. I liven them up by cooking black pepper into the whites or some chipotle pepper or, even better, scotch bonnet jerk sauce. A lot of people use salsa to make huevos rancheros. Caution: Some jerk sauces and salsa have sugars in them. Read the labels. But eggs are easy to dress up. Throw in some veggies, any kind of spice or seasoning and you have flavorful protein from a whole, unprocessed source.

Talapia is my favorite fish. I buy the frozen fillets and fry them in a pan or on a electric grill. My current favorite for seasoning Talapia is Lemon Pepper, but anything will work—just keep an eye on the salt and sugars.

My unrefined palette is at its best in restaurants. I really do not like eating out and avoid business lunches whenever possible. When I can't, I still try to be sociable and order food, but I don't use the menu.

Just about every sit-down restaurant will let you modify an order. Some places are easier than others. In the Midwest, barbecue is king, which makes life easier for me. A salad, dressing on the side, preferably Italian or just some type of vinegar and oil and a plate of meat. Barbecue sauce on the side.

In the Midwest the barbecue sauce is a tomato and sugar based. Delicious, but with my insulin reaction, a major problem. Every barbecue joint I have ever been too will gladly put the sauce on the side. Then you are able to devour a plate of smoked meat. You will be up a pound or two and a little puffy from the salt, but that goes away on its own. The sugar is something you have to work off.

I often find myself saying, "I'll have the smothered steak, but without any of the smothering—just the steak. And no glaze. Just the steak." When you say that the waiter will look at you odd for a second, but hey, they don't care—you just saved them ingredients. They will charge you full freight but only deliver three quarters of the product.

If the people I am dining with look at me odd, I just say I'm mildly allergic to whatever. I always say I'm allergic to bread. Which, given my insulin reaction to carbs and the sugars in bread, is basically true.

In that vein I'm allergic to alcohol. Beer is sugar, bourbon and whiskey have more carbs and sugars than you can imagine. A margarita or a mojito—sugar. Wine? Sugar.

If you really want a margarita, save it for part of your controlled and planned cheat and do not drink and drive—unless you want to do a metabolic reset in the county jail.

Having to navigate restaurants is a part of life. A lot of things in life can throw you off your eating plan or workouts. It is important to accept those things and do your best to keep working toward your goals.

CHAPTER THIRTY TWO
LIFE HAPPENS

Right now I have a great schedule because I own my own businesses. Most of the time I can stay in a set routine that makes it easy to train. But life still happens to me. I wind up in some war zone, or I film a TV show or run camera during a college football game.

Life will happen to all of us, it is how we respond to life that matters.

One time I had a huge project—a seven days a week, 14 hours a day project. The days were extremely arbitrary and I never new when I would be able to quit for the day. Some days I just didn't quit, I literally slept in the office.

One of the things I have found over the years is that while meetings can run long and projects to be completed can run into the night—things rarely start before 7:00 a.m.

During this project I was able to stick to a basic Phase I weight lifting rotation, pack my food and lift weights in the morning.

Yeah, getting up at 4:00 a.m. to be at the gym at 4:30 a.m. sucked, but what was the alternative? Not train? Get fat? Lose muscle? Screw that, I'll get up early a few days a week.

Before I started my own business I worked some crazy hours. At the office at 8 a.m., straight through to 5 p.m. then I had to be at the TV studio at 8:00 p.m. to do pre-production for the 10 p.m. newscast and I was still in college! Three days a week I went from work, to class to work again.

So I got up every morning and hit the gym.

I have always put in the time at the gym. Once I cracked the code and started keeping a log book and really working the overload over time, things really took off.

Everything in this book comes down to a matter of priorities. Obviously your family is the first priority. Your career, meeting your obligations are a very high priority. Your relationships are a high priority.

The decision is how are you going to position training and diet within the rankings of priority. If you put training and diet ahead of your family—you are wrong. If you put it ahead of your obligations, career and relationships—you are probably wrong.

But if going out to the bar is a higher priority than training and sticking to your eating plan, well, then you will look like going to the bar is a higher priority than training and eating right.

What is your priority. If you are starting your career, if you have bills to pay, if your family needs you—those come first. But what other things are you putting before training?

You get out of the system exactly what you put into it. If going to the lake and drinking beer is a priority for you—then don't be surprised if you have a beer belly.

Like Nita says, "The question is not whether you want to drink the beer or not, the question is 'do you want abs?'"

If you want abs, don't drink the beer outside of a controlled cheat. But as we saw in Phase II, if you really want the abs, the beer will have to go away.

NITA SPEAKS

Every choice is an investment or a cost. What you invest will determine your outcome. We all know this, but most of us seem to be missing the point.

What do you get when you say you want to be in shape, but you spend five out of seven days of your week eating pastries with coffee in the morning while drinking beer or wine every night before bed. What do you get when you spend the weekends out drinking beer and eating out indulging in fatty, starchy meals and desserts, but you eat decent during the week?

What do you get if 90 percent of the time you are staying on a well controlled eating plan and hitting the gym?

You have fallen into one of these scenarios, and thus you look and feel as you do today.

What you spent and invested of your time, energy or money has given you your current outcome. That can change. Transformation of your life comes in an instant, all in the flash second of a choice of commitment. Transformation of your body comes from constantly repeating that instant's choice of commitment to achieving your goals.

After being around Nita and a lot of competitive physique athletes I learned that while you do see them out and about on Saturday nights—it is only on occasion and that it is their controlled cheat. Remember back in Part I, when Lynnie would step out of the club to have her whey protein?

But for every guy and girl in the club with a hard body, there are 100 who are soft and flabby.

For you younger guys, especially those of you who would like to become bodybuilders, I have some advice you may never hear anywhere else—get your life established first. Get a career or a steady job. Get through college. Don't go into debt. Get yourself established first. Train of course, but treat it like a plan. It takes years to build a championship worthy physique. Poor employment, debt and the stress brought on by those will kill your efforts to build a champion physique.

The physique athletes I respect the most are the ones who have a career, or own their own businesses—who have more than their physique. If all you do is train people and basically work in a gym, how difficult is it to train and diet? If your life becomes wrapped up in the iron game, the industry, you lose perspective and your identity becomes your physique, which is not a good place to be.

My physique is a by-product of functionality. Do I enjoy it? You bet. But it is not my identity. It does not form the basis of who I am. It is just a part of who I am. I don't even wear tank tops or muscle shirts to the gym. Just a plain t-shirt and gym shorts.

If you want the physique, you have to make certain choices. Make certain things a priority. But having abs should never be a priority over paying the mortgage, taking care of your family responsibilities or meeting your obligations.

PART IV

WOMEN AND THIS SYSTEM

CHAPTER THIRTY THREE
WOMEN & WEIGHT TRAINING

My best friend and workout partner is a petite little thing named Juli. She is my gym wife—we always claim to be married and I tack her on to my membership at a reduced rate.

We just had our six year anniversary as gym partners.

Juli is not a competitor. Although she thinks she might want to do a show sometime. She is not a model, although she is gorgeous. Juli is a regular 26-year-old single girl with a career.

Juli has always admired the look of figure competitors and even women bodybuilders. But what sets her apart is that she has never been afraid of getting 'too muscular'.

Juli works out almost as intensely as I do and usually sticks to a pretty controlled eating plan. And after years of overload over time, here is a picture of her

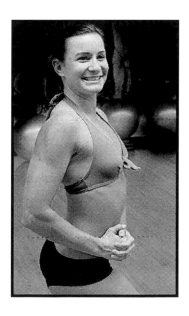

Pretty good huh?

This is a 5'3", 120 pound girl who really does Phase I all the time.

Phase I, as it turns out, is a really good bikini-body training plan for women because building muscle is the superfecta for women who want to look better in a bikini.

The Phase I workout itself burns calories. The body burns calories to repair the muscle. The muscle gain burns even more calories and fat. And, it re-shapes your body.

It is more realistic for a woman to look like a figure competitor at a local or regional competition than to look like super model or Hollywood starlet. Why? Genetics—bone structure and fat patterns.

There is no such thing as spot reduction but there is spot addition.

The three things that determine the appearance of person's physique are bone, fat and muscle.

You cannot change your bones. You can lose fat, but where you body stores fat is genetic. When you combine fat loss with building muscle—then you can start to reshape your body.

NITA SPEAKS

Lifting weights gives your body contour and tone, which is a lot more feminine than letting nature and gravity take its course. Anyone who says that lifting weights makes women look like a guy is clearly someone who just doesn't get it, and therefore, you would want to steer clear of subjecting yourself to their self-proclaimed "expertise".

A lot of women say they want to be 'toned.' But forget that muscle tone comes from muscle. Which means you have to work the muscle and overload it to tone it. Women can and should do a lot of the same exercises a guy does. They just need to adapt the frequency, volume and intensity to suit their body type and goals.

For a woman with a thick waist, she cannot make her rib cage or pelvis smaller, but she can add some width to her lats and size to her delts making her bigger on top and making her waist look smaller.

Building up the quads will also create the illusion of narrower hips. Flat butt? Build the glutes which also makes the waist look smaller.

And ladies, you will have to work just as hard, actually harder than the guys, to build the muscle.

Here is another illustration for you:

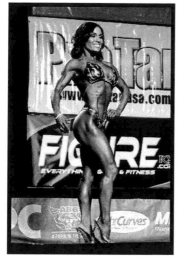
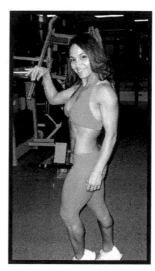
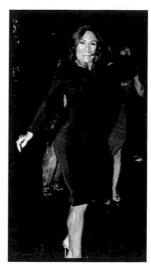

Nita
2008 NPC Jr. Nationals
photo courtesy Barry Brooks

Nita at the gym
Spring 2009

Nita out on the town

My dear friend Nita, only looks like she does in the picture on the left for one week before a contest—if even that long. Most of the time she looks like the middle picture—a great, tight, round bikini body. But if you were to see her out for a night on the town, she looks like the picture on the right, all round, firm curves.

In the chilly months of winter in Phoenix, if you saw her out and around, you would never guess she was an IFBB Professional Fitness Athlete. You would just think she is a petite woman with great curves. She's actually a petite, 35-year-old mother of three with great curves!

Weight training to build muscle is better than any diet. The ladies are more familiar with dieting than men. They seem to start doing it in high school for prom or Summer bikini season and as adults for weddings, class reunions, cruises, vacations, etc.

The problem with a traditional diet, as discussed in Phase II and Phase III is that the body adapts to the calorie restriction. The problem with diet and 30 minutes or even an hour a day on the cardio equipment is that the body adapts and then, because it becomes more efficient, burns fewer calories.

The cardio and diet will work for a few weeks or even a few months. But after that you will plateau and worse, when your body adapts, you will start to gain fat. Which is why you see so many women who put in hours on the elliptical machines that really don't look great.

But lifting weights and making protein a priority in your eating plan does work.

Now, a lot of you ladies may still not be sold. Or some of you are sold, but kind of intimidated by the weights and machines. One of the best resources is Nita's website, fitnessdirectives.com. Join for free and you will get access to a video library of how to perform nearly every exercise you will need.

But it still may be kind of intimidating to venture into the weight room.

Ladies, I have been trained by and learned more about lifting weights and diet from women than I have from men. Women taught me how to really diet to lose fat, Nita and Lisa got me doing sprints and the crazy Miami Muscle Girls taught me what real intensity in the gym is.

Get in there and mix it up with the guys—really, we're not all that bad, other than the flirting and gawking, but head phones and a baseball cap can deter a lot of that.

CHAPTER THIRTY FOUR
THE STRENGTH OF WOMEN

"What do you normally do?"

Sarah was getting ready to do a set of lat pull downs. Today was lats and traps for both of us. It was our first workout together as I took her through the system.

"70 pounds," she said.

I smiled and shook my head. "That is not enough. Try 110."

Sarah blanched. She had been doing 70 pounds for months or even years. She had never tried to go beyond it. It had never occurred to her to increase the weight, let alone jump up 40 pounds.

She looked at me skeptically, grabbed the bar and knocked off nine reps. She was surprised. I was not.

Sarah had been making a common mistake among women—not lifting heavy enough weights (men make the same mistake, but not in nearly the proportion as women.)

Over the years I've seen women carry and sling around 20 and 30 pound toddlers, then, when they go to the gym, never lift a weight over 15 pounds. A gallon of milk weighs 8.3 pounds.

Women are much stronger than they think and the laws of hypertrophy and overload overt-time apply to women just like men. In my experience, after going through Phase I, a woman can be pound-for-pound almost as strong as man. A pound of muscle is a pound of muscle whether it is on a man or a woman. Men have the benefit of DNA and higher testosterone levels to build more muscle, but the strength of a pound of muscle is uniform between the sexes.

Sarah was working the muscle for years doing lat pull downs with 70 pounds, but she was never overloading the muscle. She would squeeze the muscle and feel a lactic acid burn after a dozen reps, but never cause enough of the micro-trauma needed to build muscle and never overload the muscle frequently enough over the course of months and years.

After Sarah completed her sets of lat pull downs with 110 pounds, I did my sets with 270 pounds.

I weighed 212 pounds.   Sarah weighed 140 pounds.   Pound-for-pound, I am significantly stronger, but the pound for pound equation is thrown off by our relative levels of body fat.

For a more accurate anecdotal description we have to go Die Hard Gym in Phoenix, Arizona where Nita trains and where I train (when I'm in Phoenix).

At an offseason weight of around 110 pounds, Nita will do lat pull downs with 130 pounds.   Usually with Tim Sparkes, the owner of Die Hard and Nita's trainer of eight years, scowling over her shoulder.   Nita competes at around 100 pounds, occasionally getting as low as 97 pounds after a long stretch of contests.   But at 110 pounds, while slowly trying to add a few ounces of muscle, she still has abs.

My set of lat pulldowns is 127 percent of my body weight.   Nita's set of lat pull downs is with 118 percent.   I may be doing 140 pounds more than Nita, but I am also one-foot taller and 102 pounds heavier than Nita.

The pattern would bear out through just about every exercise.   A pound of muscle is a pound of muscle and is strong as every other pound of muscle.

The only variable is myelin tissue.   Myelin is the fatty sheath surrounding nerves that allow them to fire more efficiently.   Really athletic people tend to have more myelin than we mortals.   But, myelin tissue can be increased with practice.   This is how muscle memory works.   It works for women as well as men.   A woman who weight trains is likely to be much stronger pound for pound than a male couch potato.

If Nita, Juli, Sarah or Natasha and I were to start doing a certain exercise, over time we would all wind up moving the same percentage of weight, accounting for lean body mass as we built the muscle and became more effective at the movement.

Because of this, women should strive to train as heavy as they can which will be in a range that is proportional to men.

I'm often asked if women should train like men.   In response I usually point to Juli.

If you were to watch Nita train at Die Hard gym, her workouts are remarkably similar to what I do. Or, more precisely, my workouts are remarkably similar to hers.

My gym-wife, Juli, trains like me. I train like Nita. Nita is trained by Tim who uses the same style with her as he uses with competitive male bodybuilders.

To sum it up, Juli trains like a guy who trains like a girl who trains like a guy and it has worked out pretty good for all of us.

But some women still hesitate to lift weights hard. Their hesitation is based on two understandable fears that need to be overcome so they can quit being the female version of that guy.

CHAPTER THIRTY FIVE
THAT GIRL

There is a species of gym-goer that must be addressed in this section. For pages and pages I have told you not to be that guy who will work out hard, but not smart. He will grind out workouts, but never make any progress. His saving grace is he works out hard and keeps at it. Being *that guy* prevented me from ballooning up to a 300 pounder, saving me from my own DNA.

The gyms of the world are not only filled with *that guy* they are also populated with *that girl*.

That girl says, "I don't want to get too muscular." The key word being "too".

At first, when I heard this, I thought it was a misperception, that if women workout hard for a few weeks or months or a year they will morph into world class women bodybuilders like the Miami Muscle Girls. I would explain that it takes women bodybuilders years and years of deliberate training and often chemical enhancement to get to that level.

What I have come to find is that the misperception was not on the part of the women, but me. They knew they would never suddenly wake up being built like an extremely muscular 5'3" tall man.

The women had nothing against looking like Nita, or figure competitors or even the less muscular women bodybuilders.

I couldn't figure out what was going on when I heard women say it. So, I asked a few experts.

"Women want to be small. They want to be skinny. They want to be lean," Juli said.

Okay. That made sense. But Nita nailed it.

"Women don't want to look bulky. They would rather be plump, or skinny fat, than muscular and fat," she said.

Women don't want to look like a female version of the heavy duty guys. That makes perfect sense.

It is pretty easy for Nita to overcome these hesitations with her clients and women she encounters and to break down the fears of becoming a heavy duty girl.

The other, and more pernicious version "I don't want to get too muscular" line is a psychological defense mechanism.

It is a method of self-sabotage. An excuse to fail.

That girl likes working out. She enjoys going to the gym. She would like to look like a figure competitor or a fitness model or just a lot better than she does now, but is not sure how to do it or even if she can do it. So, she constructs an internal monologue, "I want to be in-shape, in better shape than most women, but I don't want to get too muscular."

The fear is not in becoming too muscular, the fear is in putting in a lot of effort and still failing. Even closer to the point—the fear is in a disappointment in herself. But, if she makes it okay to fail, if she makes okay to not achieve her goals, then she will not be disappointed in herself. The irrational fear of becoming too muscular is the perfect excuse to not train hard and then fail in achieving her goals.

Much in the way I built the internal monologue of how I was destined to be a heavy duty guy, or could never be lean, she builds her own internal monologue. After it is said and heard enough times, it becomes true.

To overcome the psychological self-sabotage, you must be honest. I look at pictures of the top men bodybuilders, I say to myself, "Wow." I would like to look like that, or close to it. But I am also honest with myself. I am just not willing to do what it takes to achieve it. That frees me to achieve a lesser goal. To put in the time and make the sacrifices I am willing to.

When you confront what you are willing to do and accept it, you will find that you wind up doing more to achieve your lesser goal, than you when you set yourself up for failure of the higher goal.

Remember my friend Natasha from the chapter on cardio? She kicks my ass in the gym, but even she told me that while she wanted to get leaner and more muscular than she already was, she didn't want to get too lean or too muscular.

Nita says, "If you ever get leaner than you want, or more muscular than you want, that is an easy problem to solve. Eat more fat and carbs, cut back on the training a bit." Or, more straightforward, eat some chocolate, ice cream, cheesecake and quit training for a week. Problem solved.

Natasha still has not gotten to a point of leanness and muscularity that she feels the need to ease up. I have never met a woman who intentionally quit training and started pigging out because she thought she was getting "too muscular".

The root of this psychological defense mechanism is the fear of failure. Because we are often afraid to fail, we set an incredibly high standard, determine it cannot be reached, come up with excuses why it cannot be reached and don't even try.

In terms of our own physiques, we often don't even try to achieve a lesser standard. My friend Sarah confronted this in preparation for her first figure contest.

CHAPTER THIRTY SIX
THE REAL COMPETITION

"I've been good at everything...but this," Sarah told me.

We were standing in the cardio room of the gym. She had been training and dieting for a figure contest for months and had lost twenty pounds of body fat. The definition in her quads and shoulders was starting to show. But as she stood there in a sports bra, shorts and heels, she compared herself to the women on the covers of the magazines.

Even though she was going to be doing small contest in the Midwest, and was well within the margin expected at the show, she didn't want to get on stage unless she knew she would be one of the best.

"I've been good at everything. But I'm just not good at this," she repeated.

Nita and I started working with Sarah mid-way through her contest prep. Like so many women, she was doing way too much cardio. Which in turn made it nearly impossible to make diet adjustments. But with only two months before a contest, we couldn't correct a lot the training mistakes and had to let her plow through. Hard work was not a problem for Sarah.

"When I was dieting, I never had a problem. I was never tempted, never wanted to cheat. It was my decision, why would I dislike it?" she told me recently.

But as we stood there, going through the mandatory poses, she was frustrated.

Sarah comes from a family of athletes. He parents were stand-out athletes in school, her older sister played college basketball and was a state champion track athlete. Sarah herself was a standout athlete and played basketball in college.

She grew up lifting weights and training and competing in sports. A virtuous circle kept reinforcing itself.

After college she entered the working world and is now a regional sales representative for a medical company. She always worked out a few days a week. Working out and working out hard were not Sarah's problem.

Standing there in that cardio room in front of the mirror, the problem was a fear of failure.

By any objective measure, she had already won. She looked great, a perfectly fit hour glass that would make many women say, "That's what I want to look like." Her fear was that there would be three or four girls that looked like they stepped out of a magazine showing up at the show and she would look stupid. Sarah had never failed at an athletic endeavor in her life, and the prospect of failure now frightened her.

Sarah started playing basketball shortly after she learned to walk. She was the all-star in junior high and high school. In athletic endeavors she had only known success. She always got the ribbons, medals and trophies.

A figure competition was a brand new athletic endeavor. The fear of not being the best was about to scare her out of competing.

When we first talked about competing Sarah said she wanted to do this now, before she had children. She wanted to do a few contests and see how far she could take it. She picked a small show, a starter show, almost practice. Which is how it works in bodybuilding, fitness and figure. Even IFBB Professional Nita Marquez placed sixth in her first contest—a small NPC regional in Phoenix.

"I went on-line," Sarah said, "and I looked at all those other girls, and I don't look like them."

"I don't think they are competing at this little show in Kansas," I said. She knew they weren't but wasn't buying my reasoning.

Sarah was comparing herself to the likes of Nita Marquez in 2008, when she should have been comparing herself to Nita Marquez in 1998 who placed sixth in her first contest.

My conversation with Sarah that evening mirrored one I had with a figure competitor several months before in Phoenix.

In late February 2008, Ali Stewart was just a few weeks away from her first contest. Nita had taken her through contest prep step-by-step for almost eight months. I was interviewing her as part of Nita's television series, Inside the Muscle.

Ali looked great and there was little doubt she would place in the top four at the contest but she had the same hesitation as Sarah. Ali said, "If I don't look the way I want to look, I'm not sure I can get up on stage."

For Ali, the goal was not a trophy, or a placing in a contest, the goal was physical manifestation of the picture of herself in her minds eye. The contest just provided a deadline.

Remembering those talks with Ali, I asked Sarah, "If you knew you would win this contest the way you look now, would it make you feel better about getting on stage? Is it about a trophy and placing, or is it about looking the way you want to look?"

Sarah looked at herself in the mirror. "I just don't look the way I want look. It is not about a trophy."

Curious, I asked another question, "If you could get the physique and look you want would that be enough, or would you want a trophy to validate it?"

It was about the look, not the trophy and although there was a legitimate anxiety about not being up to the standards of the contest, what really held Sarah back was that she had not achieved her goal.

I declared her the winner of the East Gym figure championships, crowned myself the men's masters champion and determined that we would take a week off from training and diet and start over from square one a week later.

The new goal was not associated with a deadline of a contest. It was to achieve the look. She would then pick a contest to do. Sarah would run through the Phases of the system in a condensed fashion.

I put her on Phase I and left for short trip to Iraq. Of course, upon my return, I was somewhat fatter and trained with Sarah a few times. She was keeping her log book and overloading over time, but she was not doing what she needed to get on a base line eating plan.

"When I made the decision to compete, I had no problems sticking to the diet," she said as we worked out. "But I just can't stop now." Sarah had gained back much of the body fat she had lost.

Our plan of getting the physique first then picking a contest wasn't working. Maybe Sarah needed the deadline.

Then I got a text message from her:

"I just had the wake up call I needed. I had a guy I know at the gym tonight ask if I had a sister named Sarah & went on to say he hadn't seen me in a while & that I 'had gotten really slim for awhile'...ouch he didn't even recognize me!!"

I do not know who Mr. Uncouth is, I would never say such a thing. Well, I might. But it got Sarah back on track.

"I used to be happy with being in the top 20 percent," Sarah said, "but then I got into the top 10 percent and really liked it. But now, I'm not in the 10 percent and want back in there and want to be in the top 5 percent. And even just for a few weeks, to be in the top 1 percent. I can't believe I traded food and beer for where I was."

The artificial and arbitrary deadline of a contest can be a great motivator for a person wanting to improve their physique, but will eventually create anxiety and leave a person unfulfilled after the contest.

The goal and the reward have to be in yourself. It has to be the look you want. Whether it is to look better in a swimsuit or look like a fitness model in a glossy magazine, the reward has to be the reflection in the mirror and the satisfaction of attaining it. The satisfaction of knowing you did all the work and have it in you to accomplish your goal is the reward.

As Nita often says, **"You are worth the work."**

CHAPTER THIRTY SEVEN
3,800 DAYS

Tiger Woods is not the best golfer in the World. Raefeal Nadal and Roger Federer, despite the rankings, are not the best Tennis Players. Jimmie Johnson and the rest of the drivers in the race for the NASCAR chase are not the best drivers.

That may sound absolutely ridiculous. Admittedly, it is, because I need to add some qualifiers.

Tiger Woods is the best golfer on the PGA tour. He is the best golfer who grew up playing golf since he was a young child. Raefeal Nadal and Roger Federer are the best mens players on the ATP tour, who also started playing tennis at a young age. Jimmie Johnson is the best NASCAR driver who also started out a young age racing motorcycles then baja style off road vehicles.

These are sports that are not often played and have peculiar points of entry. One cannot decide one day to take up stock car racing. Even if you did, you have to have thousands of hours of driving racing time to even come close to the drivers on the NASCAR circuit who often started young.

In golf and tennis, when you compare the total population of the planet to the number of people who have picked up a golf club or a tennis racquet, only a thin slice have actually had the opportunity to test even if they have an aptitude for the sport.

On the opposite end of the spectrum is soccer (futbol), in every country outside of the United States, Canada and East Asia. In the United States, the most wide open of sports is basketball.

While there are probably dozens, if not hundreds of potential unknown Tiger Woods' out there, it is a safer bet that Kobe Bryant and LeBron James really are the best.

What does this have to do with getting in shape and looking better? It goes to self-selection.

Humans tend to do things they do well. They stick with them. Consequently, they become even better at those things.

A young man who is a natural mesomorph, who is lean and muscular, is more likely to lift weights than one who is not. Moreover, the effort he puts in yields results. The positive feedback loop forms a virtuous circle. He continues to train and builds an impressive physique. He may be so naturally gifted that he can perform workouts that are nowhere near optimal for him, yet still make remarkable gains.

Others, who aspire to be like him but are less genetically predisposed, try to mimic his workouts or compare themselves to him. They do what he does, but get no results. They get discouraged. They give up or it leads to a vicious circle of trying to do the workouts that are only for the very advanced or very gifted.

Most of the personal trainers I know are predisposed to have lean muscular physiques. They gravitate towards gyms and the fitness industry. They pass on their knowledge of what works for them, and because everything works for them, their clients are getting poor advice.

Where as in golf, tennis and stock car racing, one has to use certain equipment to even begin to determine if they are pre-disposed to the sport, in competitive bodybuilding and women's figure, all that is needed is a mirror.

This leads to a self-selection process. Our naturally muscular teenage boy starts lifting weights and the virtuous circle begins. It is also where the vicious circle begins, when the person who is not so naturally inclined looks in the mirror and wants to improve the reflection. The vicious circle though, can be overcome.

Nita, my friend, business partner and co-author of this book is exact opposite of a natural for the sport she competes in—women's fitness—yet she is an IFBB professional at the pinnacle of her sport.

If Nita's DNA had its way, she would be quite the butterball. In fact, as a teenager, her nick-name was "low-fat" because she's short (4'11" on a good day) and back then checked in at 125 pounds. None of it muscle.

In fitness competitions, the athletes are judged on physical appearance, leanness and muscularity, and how well they perform a demanding fitness routine.

Nita did not have a background in gymnastics and was never formally trained in dance. She will also state rather bluntly that her bone structure is almost the opposite the one preferred by judges.

The "X" frame is preferred for men and women bodybuilders. The "Y" frame is the ideal for women's fitness and figure. The "Y" being narrow hips and waist which is determined by the distance between the iliac crests of the hips and broad shoulders being determined the distance between the acromioclavicular joints of the shoulder.

Nita is at best an "H" frame. She should have looked at herself in the mirror and said it wasn't going to work. And for years, it didn't. Even after competing at the top amateur levels for years, her frame held her back.

But bones are only one third of the element that determines the shape of the human body, the other two are fat and muscle.

Nita could not change the structure of her hips, rib cage and shoulder joints. But she could get her body fat low through very strict dieting and build up the muscles in deltoids, lats and traps.

The process took 12 years.

Or, more precisely, 12 years, two pregnancies, a torn calf, eight years with the right trainer and, most importantly, 3,800 days of making the decision to workout and eat properly.

Nita is an outlier, but only in the sense that she took her pursuit all the way to professional level.

The more typical path is similar to mine. I got my first weight set when I was in junior high. For reasons I do not know, I used it regularly and started reading the muscle magazines. By the time I was in high school I was slightly more muscular then the rest of my classmates. As you can see, the virtuous circle begins and maintains itself for years. Even though my DNA wants to me to be 300 pounds of fat, the virtuous circle kept me going as that guy and then 'heavy duty' guy, until I started to put it all together.

There are very few pure mesomorphs, but we see enough of them at the gym and enough of them go into the fitness industry that they can screw up the rest of us. There is also a lot of self-selection in the gyms and especially the free weight areas.

A lot of people I talk to in the gyms and in every day life make the mistake of comparing themselves to me the way I am now. I often hear the words, "I'll never be able to look like you, but I would like to _____." At which point I remember what the Miami Girls said when we found out about my peculiar metabolism, "You are just like Paul. You will have diet harder."

What separates Tiger Woods from the weekend duffer is his not just his innate talent, but years and years of practice. Roger Federer has thousands of hours of time with a racquet in his hands. Jimmie Johnson has been racing things with engines since he was a little kid.

What separates you from the physique you want is a little bit of knowledge, which since you have read this book you now have, and time in the gym.

Just like there are many unknown prospective Tiger's out there, but they have never picked up a golf club, there are many Nita's and JD's out there who have never really trained or ate properly for a long enough period of time.

I didn't know what I could look like. I still don't. Nita is still trying to add more size and shape to her upper body and overcome with muscle and diet, what her DNA and bones dictate.

You will not know what your physique is capable of until you start working this system and making the daily decisions to train hard, train smart, overload over time and find your eating plan and the work outs that work best for you.

CONCLUSION AND THANKS

This book has been floating around in bits and pieces for a long time and was not conceived as a book until the Summer of 2008 when I was in Phoenix shooting a TV episode with Nita.

As my physique kept improving, people at the gym would ask me for advice. So, I started typing up little things and saving them on CD-Rom to give people or email them.

With encouragement from Nita I started working on putting all those ideas into a narrative of how I found them, used them and refined the way I explained the system.

Without Nita's encouragement, this book would just be a few odd articles on message boards and on discs I kept in my gym bag.

The other great source of this book is my dear friend and gym wife, Juli. She put up with a lot of the experimental workouts during the years and has been the best workout partner a person could ever have.

Lisa Krog was a great encouragement and put up with my bouncing ideas off her.

Once I had the manuscript done, I could barely stand to read it. Jamie Borgman, an award winning television writer and magazine writer, took on the task copy editing and putting everything into a structured flow.

My friend and long-time business partner David Chavarria did the typesetting, graphics and designed the cover and back flap.

I would also like to thank Sarah & Natasha for letting me use them as examples and for trusting that the system would work—even before it was a very coherent system.

And of course, I need to thank master trainer Lynn Suave who kicked my ass and never let me slack off while I muddled through the diet and found my own eating plan.

Everything I have in life is a gift from God and all those who have helped me along the way were a blessing. In the Gospel, Jesus instructs us to bear good fruit and to be a blessing unto others. I hope this book bears good fruit in you life.

APPENDIX I: HELPFUL ARTICLES
TOOLS OF THE GYM

"If I have to tie my hands and wrists to a barbell, that is probably a sign I shouldn't be using that much weight and move on," I said to the tattooed young man.

I had just finished my sets of dumbbell rows with a 150 pound dumbbell. My hands were giving out before my back. Which is pretty common. He asked why I didn't use straps or hooks. And I gave him my philosophy. There is also a practical component as well. In Iraq and Afghanistan if I have to lift something, I'm probably not going to have straps or hooks, just my hands.

I'm often asked what kind of devices or tools I use in the gym. I always know who is likely to ask me that type of question. He is the guy who wears gloves, wrist straps, some type of claw hook tied to his writs, elbow wraps, knee wraps and a hi-tech belt and wants to know if the silver bullet solution is some gym fetish gear.

They always seem disappointed when I say I don't use any of it. I don't have anything against it. I guess it could be useful, I just don't use it most of the time.

The only gym tools in my bag right now are a three ring binder, a pen, a water bottle and my own collars. I got tired of hunting around the gym for collars to hold the weights in place so I bought my own.

If, and only if, something like power pulls makes it to the top of the rotation do I pull a belt out of the trunk of my car. That is really the only exercise where I can get up to such absurd weight that I feel the need for some hernia/lower back protection.

I've seen some serious competitive bodybuilders use all kinds of gym tools and I've seen some that don't use any. More often than not, it is that guy who is all loaded up with wraps, straps and stuff that I'm not ever sure what it is supposed to do.

If you like the wraps, straps and claws--cool, keep using them. If you are not into them, you probably don't need them.

The most important tool, the one that very few people use is the notebook.

APPENDIX I: HELPFUL ARTICLES
YOGA

Yoga. Seriously. I do yoga. I resisted yoga but Juli convinced me to do it and I really like it.

After getting pounded around in humvees, wearing body armor and having my body beaten down, yoga is part of my routine now.

A couple times a week, after my weight lifting, I'll spend five to ten minutes going through a series of yoga moves to stretch out my traps, lower back and just about every other muscle.

I don't care for most of the group classes because half the time the instructor is babbling on about lunar consciousness. My favorite instructor is a motorcycle mechanic who thinks inner peace is found with a .357 Magnum, a paper target and a box of shells.

Once I got a bunch of the poses down, I started doing them on my own.

I never would have gone into a yoga class without Juli. So guys, if you are dragging your lady friend into lift weights, return the favor and do some yoga with her. You will probably like it.

APPENDIX I: HELPFUL ARTICLES
OVERCOMING INJURIES

Inevitably you will injure something. I've never had a real bad weight lifting injury—but I have had some injuries. The worst is when I woke up on a Sunday morning and my right arm didn't work right.

At first I thought it was just the normal mild nerve pinch until I went to the gym. I knew it wasn't feeling right, so I figured I would just do some easy dumbbell benchpresses with 50 pounders.

I got them up, lowered them down and my left arm easily moved the dumbbell up. My right arm didn't move—it was stuck at chest level.

That freaked me out. My right arm is very important to me. It is my camera arm.

I tried to move my arm then found I could not flex my right pec or right tricep.

I hunted around on-line, read my anatomy book then went to my doctor, who confirmed my diagnosis—I had pinched and severely damaged my radial lateral nerve. I did it in my sleep, which evidently takes some real talent.

My doctor recommended physical therapy. I went to one session and discovered I knew what I needed to do—teach my muscle to fire again with the diminished nerve capacity.

What saved me was all those years of working out. I knew how to flex my pec and tricep. It was a long process that started with me standing in front of the mirror and just moving my arm like I would on a pec dec or cable crossover until I felt a little movement in my pec.

Same thing with my tricep.

I would have Juli stand on a bench and would get on my knees and we would use a rope doing one arm tricep extensions. At first Juli said she was only giving me less than ten pounds of resistance. Ten pounds, minus the weight of my hand and forearm is not a lot of resistance.

It took me a month of doing that and doing what I could for shoulders, lats and biceps before I could start to move weights again.

Looking back at my log book, I started over on dumbbell bench at 30 pounds. Yep, 30 pounds.

Three months later, I was back to something close to full strength. My right arm—when it comes to bench or tricep exercises is still not as strong as my left. Oh, well.

The point of this story is what I did when I was injured. I never stopped training. I did all my other workouts while rehabbing my right tricep and right pec.

You will be injured. Joints will wear out as you age.

Find a way to work around them. Work with a re-hab specialist and medical professional. Just don't give up.

APPENDIX I: HELPFUL ARTICLES
LEAN & OBESE

According the Federal Government of the United States of America, I am borderline obese.

Really, according the Body Mass Index calculator of the Centers for Disease Control & Prevention I have a BMI of 29.3. A BMI of 30 or more is considered obese.

At a height of 5'10" and weighing 204 lbs., I look like I did on the cover of this book. But, according to a bunch of really smart people I'm borderline obese.

Obviously I am not obese.

But what on earth does any of this have to with being 'Fit for Combat'?

Simple, sometimes really smart researchers and scientists have no clue what they are talking about. Buried in the fine print of all their BMI talk they do throw in this caveat, "For example, highly trained athletes may have a high BMI because of increased muscularity rather than increased body fatness."

Every month, university researchers and government researchers churn out reports on health, fitness, diet and exercise.

Just like the BMI calculator gets me totally wrong, most of these studies and reports do not apply to someone who has made it all the way to Phase III. Heck, most of them do not even apply to that guy.

My absolute favorite study, and I wish I could find it, was one that found that people who exercise in the early morning are more likely to be consistent in working out over years.

One expert then urged people to start working out in the morning.

What was the flaw in the study? The causation is not between exercising early in the morning and consistency over the years. The researcher confused correlation with causation.

There is nothing magical about working out in the morning that will make you more consistent. The causation is the people doing the exercise. People who get up early in the morning to workout tend be more dedicated to getting in their workout.

There are very few long-range, well conducted studies on people who have worked out for years.

There are thousands of researchers who swear that a, 'healthy high fiber diet' and cardio vascular exercise will help you lose weight. Yes, they will. For a few months. But they never run the experiment over the course of several years. Moreover, most of the peer reviewed studies are conducted on obese people with little or no workout history.

Years ago, when I was in the Marine Reserves while going to college, a medical student used my Platoon in a study on muscle mass, BMI and upper body strength. The first phase of the test was a disaster. The accepted protocols for testing upper body strength did not work on a group of men in their twenties who were athletic and worked out consistently—we all scored near the top percentile. The tests of upper body strength were designed for normal people, not a group of Marines. The BMI, as illustrated above, did not apply as well.

The same thing applies to most of the studies you will read about. They do not apply to someone who has been working out for a few years. They definitely do not apply to anyone who has gone through the Phases in this book. Which is why you will need to become your own one-person experiment.

In the discussion of Phase III, when I told you to experiment, and do it like a real scientist, I emphasized the need for measurement and tracking. You also need to pay attention the variables to determine causation.

If you are going to test a new eating plan, do not make any changes to your workouts. If you are going to test a new workout, do not make any changes to your diet.

If you change up your eating plan, training and cardio all at the same time, you will know the results of the overall change, but will not know which factors were the leading causes.

When you experiment with one aspect of your training or eating plan or cardio, you must keep all the other variables the same to determine its effect.

―――――――――――――― **APPENDIX II** ――――――――――――――

COLLECTION OF WORKOUTS, DIETS & CALCULATIONS

<u>Example of 'Armageddon Arm Workout'</u>
> Biceps--
> Barbell Curls x 3 Sets
> Dumbbell Curls x 3 Sets
> Machine Preacher Curls x 3 Sets
> Hammer Curls x 3 Sets
> Concentration Curls x 3 Sets

<u>Eating Plan that didn't work from when I was That Guy</u>
> Breakfast—Meal Replacement Drink
> Mid-morning—Sandwich
> Lunch—Sandwich
> Afternoon—Meal Replacement Bar
> Evening—Sandwich
> Night—Sandwich

<u>Early example of Rosenfield Principle/Overload Overtime in Action</u>

Week #1
Bench Press
235 x 8
235 x 6
235 x 3
Total Reps 17

Week #2
Bench Press
240 x 6
240 x 4
240 x 3
Total Reps 13

Week #3
Bench Press
240 x 8
240 x 5
240 x 3
Total Reps 16

Week #4
Bench Press
245 x 5
245 x 3
245 x 2
Total Reps 10

Lean Muscle Diameter Calculations

Ready for a rough application of high school geometry? And I do mean rough. There are more accurate measurements, but this will get us pretty close. Yep, we are going to use the mathematical constant of pi or 3.14.

Lets assume for a minute that your upper arm is perfect circle rather than an odd oval. This perfect circle of an upper arm is 430 millimeters (43 centimeters) in circumference, which means the diameter of the arm is 136.9 mm.

$$430/pi = diameter, 136.9 \text{ mm}$$

If the thickness of subcutaneous fat is 6 mm, the diameter of the lean tissue is 130.9.

Now, figure the lean tissue circumference.

$$C = pi \times 130.9$$

The lean circumference is 411 mm.

Using a cloth tape measure, I could determine the circumference of the outer circle. Using a pair of body fat calipers I could determine the thickness of the fat around the muscle. From there, it is geometry—Circumference divided by Pi equals diameter, subtract the thickness of fat and you know the lean tissue diameter. After a few practice runs I found it was best to do conduct these measurements with millimeters.
Back then, this is what the equation looked like:

Circumference: 394mm
Fat Thickness: 4mm

$$394/3.14 = 125.47 - 4mm = 121.47mm$$

The lean muscle diameter of my upper arm was 121.47mm. Today, as I write this, my lean muscle diameter is 137.8mm. That is a 16mm increase. That may not seem like a lot, but back then my arms were a soft 15.5 inches, now they are a leaner 17.25 inches.

Keeping track of the changes in lean muscle diameter gave me a standardized, quantifiable way to track actual muscle gains and eventually find the precise workouts and overload that worked for me. What worked for me was failure, taking the exercise to the point I could not perform another repetition.

Coach Rosenfield's Workout

This is a sample of what I did when I really started packing on muscle and strength. It came straight from Coach Rosenfield:

WORKOUT #1 UPPER BODY
      Dumbbell Shoulder Press
      Incline Bench 45 degrees
      Pull ups
      Cable Rows
      Barbell Curls
      Skull Crushers
      (Three sets of each exercise to failure)

WORKOUT #2 LOWER BODY
      Squat
      Leg Curls
      Toe Risers
      Shrugs
      Abs
      (Three sets of each exercise to failure.)

Here is what a couple weeks rotation looked like:
      Monday Workout #1
      Tuesday Low Intensity Cardio (LIC) (Treadmill 4 mph on an incline)
      Wednesday Workout #2
      Thursday LIC
      Friday Workout #1
      Saturday Off
      Sunday Off
      Monday Workout #2
      Tuesday LIC
      Wednesday Workout #1
      Thursday LIC
      Friday Workout #2
      Saturday Off
      Sunday Off
      Monday Workout #1

More advanced Rotation

I experimented with a little more advanced rotation as follows.

> Monday #1
> Tuesday LIC
> Wednesday #2
> Thursday LIC
> Friday #1
> Saturday LIC
> Sunday #2
> Monday LIC
> Tuesday #1
> Wednesday LIC
> Thursday #2
> Friday LIC
> Saturday #1
> Sunday LIC
> Monday #2
> Tuesday Off
> Wednesday Off
> Thursday #1
> (Repeat the Pattern)

3 Exercises 3 Times a week rotation

> Monday Workout #1 Upper Push
> Shoulder Press
> Bench
> Skull Crushers
> (Three sets to failure.)

Wednesday Workout #2 Legs

> Squat
> Leg Curls
> Toe risers
> (Three sets to failure.)

Friday Workout #3

> Lat Pull downs
> Barbell Curls
> Shrugs
> (Three sets to failure.)

1st Pre Iraq workout

My workout rotation in preparation for that first trip to Iraq started like this:

    Monday—Weights
    Tuesday—Walking/Running
    Wednesday—Weights
    Thursday—Walking/Running
    Friday—Weights
    Saturday—Walking/Running
    Sunday—Off

More advanced pre-Iraq workout from 2005
As the time for me to head to Iraq got closer, I increased the load:

    Sunday—AM Walking
            PM Weights
    Monday—Running/Walking
    Tuesday—AM Walking
            PM Weights
    Wednesday—Running/Walking
    Thursday—AM Walking
            PM Weights
    Friday—Off
    Saturday—Sprints

My weight training was the basic three day workout:

    Sunday--Upper Body Push
    Tuesday--Legs, kinda light though due to all the running
    Thursday--Upper Body Pull

Diet from when I first started trying to lose fat *that didn't work*

       Whey Protein shake with Almond Milk
       Power Walk
       Meal #1 Meal replacement shake
       Meal #2 Steak, sweet potatoes, veggies
       Meal #3 Meal replacement shake
       Lift weights or Sprints/Plyo/Agility
       Meal #4 Meal replacement shake
       Meal #5 Chicken, sweet potatoes, veggies
       Meal #6 Steak or Chicken, sweet potatoes, veggies
       Meal #7 Whey protein drink

Sample of Heavy Duty Diet Calculated

Here's a look at my heavy duty diet in the hours leading up to my weight lifting.

6:00 a.m. Wake up

Whey Protein Drink
150 Cal
27 g Protein
2 g carbs

Glutamine caps

Cardio--
Run on treadmill @ 6.5 mph then walk 4 mph 1% incline

7:30 a.m.
Meal Replacement Drink
350 Cal
32 g Protein
12 g Carbs
With a tablespoon of flax oil

9:45 a.m.
5 Jumbo eggs with cheese (5 whites, 1 Yolk) and 14 g cheese
155 Cal
30.5 g Protein
3 g carbs

11:00 a.m.
Chicken meal
150 g of charcoal grilled chicken breast
75 g sweet potato
35 g broccoli
14 g cheese

390 Calories
45 g protein
16.75 g carbs

12:00
Meal Replacement Drink
350 cal
32 g protein
12 g carbs

1:00 Lift weights M, W, F Run sprints, plymetrics, agility T, Th

Phase I Step 1 Workouts

Day One
Workout #1
CHEST PRESS MACHINE (Any kind)
SHOULDER PRESS MACHINE (Any kind)
TRICEP PUSH DOWNS (Straight or slightly angled bar)

Day Two
Off or Short Duration Sprints

Day Three
Workout #2
LEG PRESS
LEG CURLS
CALVES (any exercise)

Day Four
Off

Day Five
Workout # 3
LAT PULL DOWNS (any grip)
BARBELL CURLS (straight or EZ)
SHRUGS (Any kind)

Day Six
Off or Short Duration Sprints

Day Seven
Off

Phase I Step 2 Option B Workout

In Option B, things get shook up a little bit more as the frequency is increased.

Here's an Option B workout:

Workout #1
Barbell or Dumbbell Bench Press
Barbell or Dumbbell Shoulder Press
Barbell Rows or Power Pulls
Wide Grip Skull Crushers or Bench Dips
Shrugs of any kind

Workout #2
Barbell or Dumbbell curls
Squats or Any kind of leg press
Leg Curls of any kind
Toe risers of any kind

Option B Rotation
Day One
Workout #1

Day Two
Off or Short Duration Sprints

Day Three
Workout #2

Day Four
Off

Day Five
Workout #1

Day Six
Off or Short Duration Sprints

Day Seven
Off

Day One
Workout #2

Day Two
Off

Day Three
Workout #1

Day Four
Off or Short Duration Sprints

Day Five
Workout #2

Example of JD's current eating plan calculated

Write yours out so it looks something like my current eating plan below:

Training & Diet
Protein 315 grams
Carbs 64 grams
Sugar 10 grams

3:00 a.m. (midnight snack if I wake up hungry)
Whey protein shake with water
18 Grams protein
2 grams sugar

6:00 a.m.
Whey Protein shake with water, 1 Amino Acid Tab, 2 Glutamine Caps
18 Grams Protein
2 Grams Sugar

6:30 a.m. Sprints

7:00 a.m.
1 Cup Oatmeal (80 grams) with two scoops whey powder and Flax Oil
20 Grams Protein
52 Grams Carbohydrate
4 Grams Sugar

9:30 a.m.
8 Egg whites, 3 yolk
33g Protein
2g carbs

12:00 p.m.
Steak meal with broccoli
170 grams steak
315 Cal
45g protein
3g carbs
1 Amino Acid Tab, 2 Glutamine Caps

1:00 p.m. Lift Weights

2:30 p.m. Whey Protein Shake 2 scoops
36 Grams Protein
4 Grams Sugar

4:30 p.m.
8 Egg whites, 3 yolk
155 Cal
33g Protein
2g carbs

7:00 p.m.
8 Egg whites, 3 yolk
155 Cal
33g Protein
2g carbs

9:00 p.m.
170 grams steak
45g protein
1 Amino Acid Tab, 2 Glutamine Caps

10:00 p.m.
Go to Bed

On Wednesday, I eat a huge green salad

Saturday, I do a crazy cheat eating all kinds of crap

JD's Heavy Duty Eating plan calculated

6:00 a.m.
Wake up
Whey Protein Drink
150 Cal
27 g Protein
2 g carbs
Glutamine caps

6:30 a.m.
Cardio

7:30 a.m.
Meal Replacement Drink--
350 Cal
32 g Protein
12 g Carbs
With Flax oil

9:45 a.m.
5 Jumbo eggs with cheese
5 whites, 1 Yolk
155 Cal
27 g Protein
2 g carbs
14 g cheese
3.5 g protein
1 g carb

11:00 a.m.
Chicken meal
150 g charcoal grilled chicken breast
75 g sweet potato
35 g broccoli
14 g cheese
390 Calories
45 g protein
16.75 g carbs

12:00 p.m.
Meal Replacement Drink
350 cal
32 g protein

12 g carbs
1:00 p.m.
Lift weights

2:30 p.m.
Meal Replacement Drink
350 Cal
32 g Protein
12 g carbs
Glutamine caps

4:00 p.m.
Chicken meal
150 g charcoal grilled chicken breast
75 g sweet potato
35 g broccoli
14 g cheese
390 Calories
45 g protein
16.75 g carbs

6:30 p.m.
chicken meal
150 g charcoal grilled chicken breast
75 g sweet potato
35 g broccoli
14 g cheese

9:00 p.m.
another chicken meal

10:00 p.m.
Go to bed

3:00 a.m.
"Midnight" snack
Whey protein
150 Cal
27 g Protein
2 g carbs

Total Per Day
Protein 357 g
Carbs 120 g

The ketogenic carb cycle

Day 1 Saturday—
Your cheat meal should be down to some extra oatmeal and a salad and do what you normally do on Saturday.

Day 2 Sunday—
No carbs, no sugars. Replace any remaining carbs with a protein source of equal calories. You will feel like crap today.

Day 3 Monday—
Same as Sunday.

Day 4 Tuesday—
Same as Monday

Day 5 Wednesday—
Eat the same as Tuesday. Use your keto strips a few times during the day. Did they turn color? Are you Ketogenic? Some people will be ketogenic by now. Some will not.

Day 6 Thursday—
Eat the same as Wednesday. Use your keto strips. Most everyone will be getting some ketones in their system by now. Many of you will start to feel better.

Day 7 Friday—
Same as Thursday.

Day 8 Saturday—
Same as Friday, but if you want to have a ketogenic cheat day, give it a shot. How do you have ketogenic cheat day? By eating a lot of fat, like Pork Rinds, bacon, sausage, etc. Be careful on the sausage as many types contain sugars. The ketogenic cheat day breaks the monotony of the eating plan and keeps the body from adapting to the relatively constant caloric intake.

Day 9 Sunday—
Back on the usual ketogenic diet. If you did the cheat, your keto strips test will show a higher concentration of ketones.

Day 10 Monday—
Same as Sunday

Day 11 Tuesday—
Same as Monday

Day 12 Wednesday—
You can have carbs again in the manner listed below for the next 48 hours

You will be eating every two hours for the next 48 hours. The closer you can get to eating every two hours the better. *Really, get up in the middle of the night and eat.*

Here is what your carb re-feed plan should look like:

Meals 1-4:	Fruit juice with whey protein, a big glass of it
Meals 5-9:	50% Fruit juice, 50% water with whey protein in the big glass
	Some type of breakfast cereal made from corn
Meals 10-14	Steak, sweet potatoes, vegetables, oatmeal and a shot of fruit juice
Meals 15-18	Steak, sweet potatoes, vegetables, oatmeal, pasta, no fruit juice
Meals 19-24	25% fruit juice, 75% water with whey protein in the big glass

Then you repeat the cycle starting at the second day with no carbs.

A Phase III type Pattern

Monday
AM Sprints
PM Weights

Tuesday
AM Sprints
PM Weights

Wednesday
AM Nothing
PM Weights

Thursday
Off or functional distance

Friday
AM Sprints
PM Weights

Saturday
AM Easy Intervals, Agility or Nothing
PM Weights

Sunday—Off

Phase III Sample Workout

Monday
AM Sprints
PM Standing Dumbbell Shoulder Press 3 sets
　　　Machine Lateral Raises 3 sets
　　　Leaning Single Arm Side Laterals 2 sets

Tuesday
AM Sprints
PM Hack Squat 2 sets
　　　Lying Leg Curls 2 sets
　　　Toe risers 2 sets

Wednesday
> AM Nothing
> PM Wide Grip Lat Pull downs 3 sets
> > Machine Row 3 sets
> > Machine Rear Delt Flys 2 sets
> > Smith Machine Shrugs 2 sets

Thursday
> Off

Friday
> AM Sprints
> PM Barbell Flat Bench Press 3 sets
> > Machine Incline 3 sets

Saturday
> AM Easy Interval Running and/or Agility
> PM Tricep Extensions 3 sets
> > Barbell Curls 3 sets
> > Skull Crushers, wide grip 3 sets
> > Dumbbell Curls 2 sets each arm

Sunday—Off

Phase III Sprints Rotation
> Monday AM
> Sprints
>
> Tuesday AM
> Sprints
>
> Wednesday AM
> None
>
> Thursday AM
> None/or Functional Distance
>
> Friday AM
> Sprints

Saturday AM
None/or Easy Interval/or Agility Drills

Sunday AM—None

—————————————————— **APPENDIX III** ——————————————————

JULY 28, 2008 THROUGH OCTOBER 15, 2008

PM 204.2 lbs   Mon July 28

   An sprinst   50x5

Cable side Lateral
70x   Left   Right
        7   7
        3.5   3.5
        2   2

Cable upright (27)
160x 13   w
       6   N
       4   w
       4   N

DB Incline   (20)
80x 14   450
     4   650
     2   800

~~Arnold~~ Shoulder Press DBell (15)
         7
   50x   3
      X
      X 2

Bench side Laterals
70x   Right   Left
       11   11
        6   6
        4   4

203.4   Tuesday July 29

      AM Sprints

    Leg ext
    150 x 20   Straight
        12   Toe in
        9   Toe Out

    Single Leg Curls
      Right   Left
60x   10   10
      5   6
      3   3

    Walking Lunges
      60x   prt

    Toe risers
    105 x 17

203.0   Wed July 30

AM none

DB Rows
Left   Right
100x   9   9
          5   5
          4   4

Cable Rows
210x   8
x   4
x   3
drop150x 4

DB Rear Delts
20x   13   forward
          6   down

66 Pulls
225x   10
x   3.5
x   2
drop 165 x   4

202.4 Lbs   Friday Aug 1
                     AM Sprints 10x50 10 min

Cable Crossover (20)
    100 x 12
        x 5
        x 3

DB Flat   13 ?
    90 x 8
       x 3
       x 2

DB Incline 45° 12.5
    75 x 6
       x 3.5
       x 3 + Flail

Machine Incline (20)
    180 x 13
        x 5
        x 2

2028   Sat Aug 2   Up Late
                                  Sat night

AM none

Rope Ext (14)
90 x 8
   x 3
   x 3

BB Curls   Done!
145 x 12
    x 2
    x 3

W6 Skull Crushers (19)
90 x 11
   x 5
   x 3

DB Preacher
        Right   Left
40 x   12   12
   x   4   4
   x   2   2

~~One arm Dumbell Overhead~~
~~Right~~

Bench Dips Ball
10 x 23
   x 8
   x 6

206.0   Mon Aug 4th

Sprints 11x50 10mm

Cable Side Lateral

	Right	Left
70x	34	9
	5.5	5.5
	3.5	3.5

Cable upright   34

160x 18   w
9   w
5   w
4   w

DB Incline   14
85 x 7   45°
34   60°
3   75

DB Shoulder Press   18
50x 11
4
3

Bench Side Laterals

	Left	Right
25x	5	5
	3	3
	1	1

204.4   Tue Aug 5
AM spints
12 x 50 10 mm

Leg ext
165 x 19   Straight
    x 8   Out
    x 5   M

single Leg curls
         Left   Right
60 x   13   13
    x   6   6
    x   4   4

walking Lunges
70 60 x   1 RT

Seated Toe Risers
105 x 21

203.4   Wed Aug 6
                    AMnone

        DBRows
              Right   Left
    110×   11   11
              5   5
              3   3

        Cable Rows   (17)
        210 × 11
            × 4
            × 2
    Drop 150 × 6

        Rear Delts
        20× 14.5   T down
            8.5 †Flails T forward

        66 Palls   Done!
    225 × 9
        × 4
        × 2.5
    drop 165 × 3

        Shrugs
        85×12 Bent
            5 straght

2024   Friday Aug 8
              AM Sprints

Cable Crossovers (12)
110 × 7
    × 3
    × 2 + Flails

DB Flat   (18)
90× 12
   × 4
   × 2

DB Incline 45° 13
75 × 6
   × 4.5
   × 3 + flails

Machine Incline
145 × 9 + Flails
    × 4 × Flails
    × 2 + Flails

Harley Party Coke
2 diet coke
Baby Chicken

205   Sat Aug 9th

        AM none hurt groin Friday

    Rope Ext   (16)
      90 × 10
          × 4
        × 2 + 1 Flail

    W 6 Skull Crushers
      100 × 6
          × 3
        × 2 + Flail

    DB Preacher
        Right   Left
  45×   6   6
    ×   3   3
    ×   3   3

    Bench Dips Ball
    25 × 22
       × 4
       × 6

    Dumbell curls (20)
      50 × 11
         × 5
         × 4 + Flail

206   Monday 11   Start Keto

AM 5 min sprints

Cable Side Laterals
           Left   Right
70x   10.5   13.5
  x   6.5   6.5
  x   4.5   4.5

Cable Upright   (19)
170x 7   W
      5   N
      4   W
      3   N

DB Incline   (18)
85 x 10   45
     4   ~~50~~ 45°
     2   ~~50~~ ~~25°~~ 75°

DB Shoulder Press (10)
55 x 6
   x 2
   x 2

      Bench Side Laterals
           Right   Left
25x   7   7
         3   3
         2   2

204.2   The Aug 12   Ketogenic

AM 7min strides

Leg ex 4
16-5 X 24   Straight
      11   M
      8   out

Single leg Curls
    Right   Left
60x   15   15
     6   6
     4   4

Seated Toe r310
135X 13
   X 8

2038   Wed Aug 13   Ketosis
                                                d Leg
                    Ah none

            DB Rows
              Left   Right
    120x   7   5
              3   4
              2.5   3.5

        Cable Rows
        225 X 7
            X 2
            X 2
    drop 165 X 4

        Rear Delts
    25 x 10   T forward
          9   T down

    Wide Grip Pulldowns Front
    180 x 9
        X 2
        X 2

    Shrugs
    85 x 10
        X 8

Fri Aug 15th   Ketosis
AM none
Cable crossovers (17)
110× 11
    × 4
    × 2+ Flails

DB Flat   (10)
95× 6
    × 2+ Flails
    × 2+ Flail

DB Incline 45°   (14)
75× 7.5
    × 4+ Flail
    × 3.5 +Flail

Machine Incline   (18)
195× ~~15~~ 10
    × 5
    × 3+Flails

Sat Aug16th   Ketosis
AM none
Rope ext   (18)
90 × 11
  × 4 + Flail
  × 3 + Flail

W6 Skull Crushers (13)
100 × 8
   × 3.5
   × 2 + Flails

DB Preacher
      Left   Right
45 × 8   8
   × 5   5
   × 4   4

Bench Dips Ball
35 × 18
   × 7
   × 4

Dambell Curls (14)
55 × 8 & 4
   × 4
   × 2 + Flails

203.8   Mon Aug 18th   Ketosis

AM none

Cable Side Lateras

        Right   Left
89 X   4.5   4.5
   X   2.5   2.5
   X   1.5   1.5

    Cable Upright   w (31)
170 X 13   N
    X 8   N
    X 6   w
    X 4   N

DB Incline   (19)
85 x 12   45°
   X 5   65°
   X 2 + Flail 75°

DB Shoulder press (14)
55 X 8
   X 4
   X 2 + Flail

    Bench Side Lateral
        Left   Right
25 X   9   9
   X   6   6
   X   3   2

201.2   Tue Aug 19   Ketosis
                                                early AM gis

        Leg ext
        180 X 20   Straight
            X 8   out
            X 6   in

        Single leg curls
           Left   Right
    70 X   9   9
       X   4   4
       X   3   3

        Toe Risers
        135 X 18
            X   9

201.4   Wed Aug 20   Ketosis

AM none

DB Rows
         Right   Left
120 x   18   10
     x   4.5   4.5
     x   3   3

Cable Rows
   125 x   9
        x   2
        x   2
drop 165 x 2 +Flails

Rear Delts
30 x   5.5   ↑ Down
    x   5.5   ↑ Forward

Undergrip Pulldowns Front
   180 x   12
        x   5
        x   3

Shrugs
  40 x   9   Bent
       x   7   Straight

200.8   Fri Aug 22

AM None

Cable Crossovers (20)
110 × 13
    × 5
    × 2

DB Flat   (15)
95 × 10.5
    × 3. Fail
    × 2. Flail

DB Incline   Done!
75 × 6.5
    × 3
    × 2 + Flails

Machine Incline (20)
195 × 12
    × 5
    × 3, 5 + Flail

202   Sat Aug 23rd   Basediet
             AM none

Rope ext (19)
90 × 12
   × 4
   × 3

W/6 skull crushers (16)
100 × 9
    × 5
    × 2

DB Preacher
        Right   Left
45 ×   9   9
   ×   5   5
   ×   3   3

Bench Dips Ball
45 × 23
   × 9
   ×

Dumbbell Curls
55 × 10
   × 5
   × 3.5 + F [ails]

Stretch

295.6   Mon Aug 25th   Basdiet
          AM 5x50 5min

Cable Side Laterals
        Left   Right
80x   6.5   6.5
 x   4.5   4.5
 x   2+Fail   2+Fail

Cable Upright   (21)
189x   7   W
  x   5   N
  x   5   N
  x   4   N

DB Incline   (18)
90x   9   45 0
  x   6   65 0
  x   3   80 0

DB Shoulder   (16)
55x   10
  x   4
  x   2.5

Bench Side Lateral
      Right   Left
25x   10   10
  x   6   6
  x   5   5

203Lbs   Tue Aug 26
               AM 6 x 50 Loops 5 min

    Leg ext
        180 x 22   Straight
             8   M
             7   Out

    Single Leg curls
         Right   Left
70x   11   11
  X   5   5
  X   3   3

    Toe Rises
       135 x
           X

203.2   Wed 27th   Stayed up
                                  too late
        An none   feel like
                                  shit

        DB Rows
          Left   Right
130 x   5   5
    x   3   3
    x   3   2

        Cable Rows (15)
        225 x 11
            x 3.5
            x 1.5
drop 165 x 4

        Rear Delts
        30 x 12   T forward
             4   T Down

    Wide Grip Pulldowns
        180 x
            x
            x

    Shrugs
      90 x   Bent
                  Straight

201.2   Fri Aug 29th

AM   6x50 Loops

Cable Crossovers   <u>Panel</u>

120 X 4

X Flail

X Flail

DB Flat   (19)

95 X 13

X 4

X 2

Machine Incline (21)

210 X 11

X 6

X 4

Stability Ball Pushups

X 8

X 6

201.8   Sat Aug 30th

AM none

Rope ext   (9)
100 x 4 + flail
    x 3 + Flail
    x 2 + Flail

WG Skull Crushers (18)
100 x ||
    x 4
    x 3

DB Preacher   (20)
       Left   Right
45 x   10   10
   x   6   6
   x   4   4

        Bench ~~DB's Batt~~   DBell Tricarm
        ~~70 x~~   overhead
          x   60 x 12
                                x   4
Dumbell Curls (12)   x   4
  60 x   6
     x   4
     x   2

205.6   Mansept I   LS sore
                                  w/pain+
               AM 7x50 6mm   something else
                                  in trap
Cable Side Laterals
        Right   Left
80x   8   8
  x   5   5
  x   3+Flails   3+Flails

        Cable Upright   (31)
150x   12   w
  x   8   w
  x   6   w
  x   5   w

DB Incline (21)
     90x   13   45 0
       x   5   65 0
       x   3   85 0

DB Shoulder
  55x   11   Langrest talked to Rady
    x   12
    x   3

Bench Side Lateral
        Left   Right
30x   3   3
  x   2   2
  x   1   1

204   Tue Sep+2
          AM 8×50 6min

          Leg ext
          180×25   Straight
              ×18   Out
              ×8   M

          Single Leg Curls
              Left   Right
          80×   8   8
            ×   4   4
            ×   3   3

   Sms Toe risers   Left   Right
          BW×   24   24
             ×

2024   Wed Sept 3

DB Rows

~~115~~
130x   Right   Left
   x   8   8
   ~~x~~   5   5
      3   3

Cable Rows (16) ?
225 x 10
     x 4
     x 2
Drop 165   x 4 + Flails

    Rear Delts
30 x 14   T Down
   x 5   T Forward

Wide Grip Pulldowns Front (17)
180 x 3
    x 2
    x 2

Shrugs
90 x 13   Bent
    9   Straight

2028   Fri Sept 5th   Korean Cheat meal
                                        Thursday
            AM sprints 8x50 6mm

DB Flat   (18)
    100 x 11
        x 5
        x 2.5

    Machine Incline   (16)
    225 x 11
        x 3 + Flais
        x 2 + Flails

    Incline DB Flys 45° (15)
        30 x 9
           x 4
           x 2

    Stability Ball Push ups
            x 12
            x 11

205.2   Mon Sept. 8th   Took
                                      sat off

          AM 98x50 7min

        Cable Side Laterals
           Left   Right
      80x   10   18
        x   6   6
        x   4   4

          Cable upright
      190 x 8   W
          x 6   W
          x 6   W
          x 3   W

        DB Incline
      95 x 12   45⁰
         x   3   65⁰
         x   2   80⁰

        DB Shoulder
      60x   8
        x   2
        x   2

        Bench Side Lateral
           Right   Left
      30x   4   4
        x   3   3
        x   1   1

203.6   Tue Sept. 9th
                    AMSpnts
          Leg ext
          180 × 27 _____ Straight
              X   in
              X   _____ out

          Single Leg Curls
              Right   Left
          80 × 11 _____ 11
              X
              X

          Single Toe Risers
              Right   Left
          Bw × 25   25
              X

204   Wed Sept. 10   Did
           AM none   Radiou/Megan

DB Row
        Left   Right
130x
   x   6   6
   x   4   4
         3   3

→ ~~Cable Rows~~ Done
  ~~225 x~~
    ~~x~~
    ~~x~~
~~Drop 165 x~~

        Rear Delts
39x 16   T Forward
  x 6   T Down

        Wide Grip Pulldowns (21)
190   x   1   5
      x   5
      x   4

    Shrugs
95x 11   Bent
   x 7   Straight

202.8   Fri Sept 12   Didall
                                              Julis
                                              Flea Laundry
         DB Flat (15)   working
         110 x 10
             x 3
             x 2
         4th x 2 Forced
         Machine Incline (28)
         225 x 15   talk w/ Sarah
             x 10
             x 3

         Incline DB Flys (25)
            30 x 15
               x 6
               x 4

         Stability Ball pushusp
              x 14
              x 9

2028   Sat Sept 13

AM Sprints

Rope Ext   (10)

4   100 × 6
3   × 3
2   × 1 + Flails

W6 Skull Crushers (9)
    110 × 5
        × 2 + Flails
        × 2 + Flails

DB Preacher
        Right   Left
    50 ×   5   5
        × 3   3
        × 2   2

Dumbell Carls (14)

6   60 × 7
4   × 4
2   × 3

201.4   Monday Sept. 15   Worked out
                                        Late
               Am sprints   Trained Theresa

PM

Cable side Laterals
      Right   Left
90x 4   4
   x 1   1
   x 1   1

      Cable upright   26
190x 13   W
    x 8   W
    x 3   W
    x 2   W

DB incline ?
95 x 13
   x 3
   x 3

DB shoulder
60x 2   3
   x   3
   x   2

Bench side Lateral
      Left   Right
39 x
   x
   x

201.4   Tues Sept. 16
       AM 12x50 8min

Leg ext
180 x 2 5   Straight   Done!
       11   M
       8   Out

Single Leg Curls   Done!
       Left   Right
80x   11   10
  X   3   2.5
  X   3   5

Single Toe rises
       Left   Right
Bwx   8   8
   X   16   16

199.8   Wed Sept 17   Lower?
        AM none   food, fucked
                                                up eating plan
    PM
    DB Row
          Right   Left
139x   9   9
    x   4   4
    x   3

    Wide Grip Pulldowns
    210 x 9
        x 2
        x 1   + Flails

    Rear Delts
    35 x   5   T Down
           4   T Forward

    Shrugs
    95 x 12   Bent
          9   Straight

200.4   Fri sept 19

DB Flay (18)
110 x 11
X 5
X 2

Machine Incline (13)
240 x 8
X 3
X 2

Incline DB Flys (11)
35 x 6
X 3
X 2

Stability Ball Pushup
X LOT
X LOT

200   Sat Sep 20
                        All Sprints #50x139min

Rope ext.   (13)
100X 8.5
    X 3
    X 2

W6 Skull Crushers (10)
110X 7
    X 3
    X 2

DB Preacher
      Left   Right
50X   6   6
   X   4   4
   X   1   1

Dumbell Curls (15)
60X   8
   X   4
   X   3

202　　　　Mon Sep 22
　　　　　Am Sprints
　　　　　　50 x 13　9 min

Cable Side Laterals
　　　　Left　　　Right
99x　　2　　　　2
　　　2　　　　2
　　　1　　　　1

Cable Upright (32)
119x　12 14　　W
　　　1　　　　W
　　　4　　　　W
　　　3　　　　W

DB Incline (14)
100 x　2
　　x　4
　　x　2

DB Shoulder (17)
60 x　2
　x　4
　x　2

Bench Side Lateral　　Done!
　　　Left　　Right
50x　4　　　4
　x　2　　　2
　x　1　　　1

202.4   Tue Sept 23   Late,
                    Sprints   MKC.
                    50×14 10 mn   during day

            Seated Leg Press
            150 × 20
                    × 15
                    × 13

            Lying Leg Curls
            75 × 14
                    × 5
                    × 3

            Toe Rises
            B   Right   Left
            BWK 22   24
                    × 16   17

            Abs
            Stretching

200.4   Wed Sept 24

        All none

    DBRow   (19)
        Left   Right   (Need Claws/wraps)
130x 10   9
    x   5   5
    x   4   4

    Wide Grip Pulldowns
        210x 11
          x   3
          x   2

    Rear Delts
    35x 11   ↑Forward
               ↑Down

    Shrugs
    95x 11   Bent
          5   straight

200.4   Fri Sept 26
             All none

DB Flat   (11)
120 x 4 5
      x 4
      x 2

Machine Incline (19)
240 x 11
      x 5
      x 3

Incline Flys (15)
35 x ø8
      x 4
      x 3

Stability Ball Pushups
Bw x 9
      x 4
(Feet in Bosu ball)

201   Sat Sept. 27
            AM 10x70 strides 10mm

Rope ext   Done!
160 x 8.5
     x 7
     x 7

W6 Skull Crush (14)
110 x 8
     x 4
     x 2

DB Preacher   Done!
    Right   Left
50 x 6   6
   x 3   3
   x 2   2

DB Curls (16)
60 x 4
   x 4
   x 3

203   Wed Oct 1   Sore Throat
                            Pase for days

AM none
~~Machine Shoulder~~

DB Incline
100 × 8
      × 7

DB Shoulder
60 × 8
   × 6

Tricep ext Rope
100 × 2
    × 2
80 × 2

203.6   Mon Oct 6   Back
                                  From cold

              AM Sprints
              ~~~~~~~~ 10 x 508 mm

Cable Side Laterals
       Right   Left
90x   6   6
  x   3   3
  x   2   2

Cable Upright Rows (Flex Fitness)
190 x 15   W
    x   9   W
    x   4   W
    x   3   W   (Did something
                        2 my right hand)

DB Incline   45°
100 x 8   60°
    x 5   60°
    x 1   80°

DB Shoulder
65 x   6
   x   2
   x   2

2014   Tue Oct 7

AM Sprints
10 × 50 8 min

DB Row
Right Left
140 ~~~~ × 3   4
       × 4   4
       × 2   2

Wide Grip Pulldowns (19)
210 × 13
    × 4
    × 2

Rear Delts
35 × 6   T Down
   × 7   T Forward

Shrugs
45 × 12   Bent
   × 8   Straight

200.0   Wed Oct 8

AM none

DB Flat
120 X 7   (14)
    X 4
    X 3

Machine Incline (18)
255 X 12
    X 4
    X 2

Incline flys
35 X 11
   X 5
   X 3

Stability Ball Pushups (Feet on Bosu)
/2

200.0   Thu Oct 9

AM 10mm KickStrides

WG Skull Crushers (18)
110 × 12
     × 2
     × 3

DB Curls (18)
60 × 11
   × 4
   × 3

One Arm DB Overhead
~~30~~   Right   Left
30 ×   10   12
   ×   4   5
   ×   3   3

Cable Curls
90 × 24   ✓
   × 10   N
   ×   W

205   Mon Oct 13   Huge TX
                                  cheat

AM spines
12x50 10mm

Cable Side Laterals
       Left   Right
90x   3   4
 x   4   4
 x   1   2

Cable Upright Raw
200 x 10   W
     x 7   W
     x 4   W
     x 4   W

DB Incline
100x13   45°
   x 3   60°
   x 1   80°

DB shoulder
65 x 3
   x 3
   x 2

203.6   Wed Oct 15
             AM none

DB Rows
        Left   Right
140x   6.5   6
   x   4   3
   x   2   2.5

Wide Grip Pulldowns
   225x   7.5
      x   3.5 Flails
      x   1.5 Flails

Rear Delts
   35x 12+Flails T Forward
       4+ Flail T Down

Shrugs
   95x 13   Bent
        11   Straight